# LIFE AFTER 50

# LIFE AFTER 50

OSMAN FATİH GÜNER

ISBN: 979-8-9865139-0-4

First Printing, 2022

# CONTENTS

## EPILOGUE 209

To my father... with whom I too early lost my chance to have an adult relationship

# ACKNOWLEDGEMENT

I would like to acknowledge the people who assisted with the creation of this memoir. Donald Wise conducted an editorial assessment. Michael Sanders provided developmental editing and copy editing. Jennifer Stimson designed the cover. Lisa Balbes wrote the back cover copy.

In addition, Kurt Güner, Sibel Güner, and Michele Larkin carried out critical review of the manuscript; and Lise Dumont performed the final line-editing and read through.

# Preface

This memoir is the story of how my professional life in the United States—its successes and failures—helped me evolve into a more peaceful and self-aware person.

I'm currently residing in Turkey having recently moved here from the US. I was born in Turkey in 1956 and went through my primary school education here. I received my BS in chemistry and MS in organic chemistry here as well. In 1982, I moved to the US to get my PhD and ended up staying there for thirty-nine years until 2021.

From 1996-2005, I worked at Accelrys, Inc., a leading company in molecular modeling and computational chemistry. I managed the company's chemistry products, which were about a third of the overall business.

\* \* \*

A few months before my fiftieth birthday, in September 2005, Accelrys laid me off, which resulted in a dramatic change in my career and in my approach to life.

This memoir also reflects on my struggle to come to terms with this change: My *Life After 50*.

## Disclaimer

This book reflects on my personal memories of events in my life. I recognize that some people mentioned may have different recollections and hence may disagree with depictions of events. Names, descriptions, and locations of some people were changed to protect the privacy of the individuals mentioned. This book was not intended to hurt anyone; both my publisher and I regret any unintentional harm that may result from the publishing of *Life After 50*.

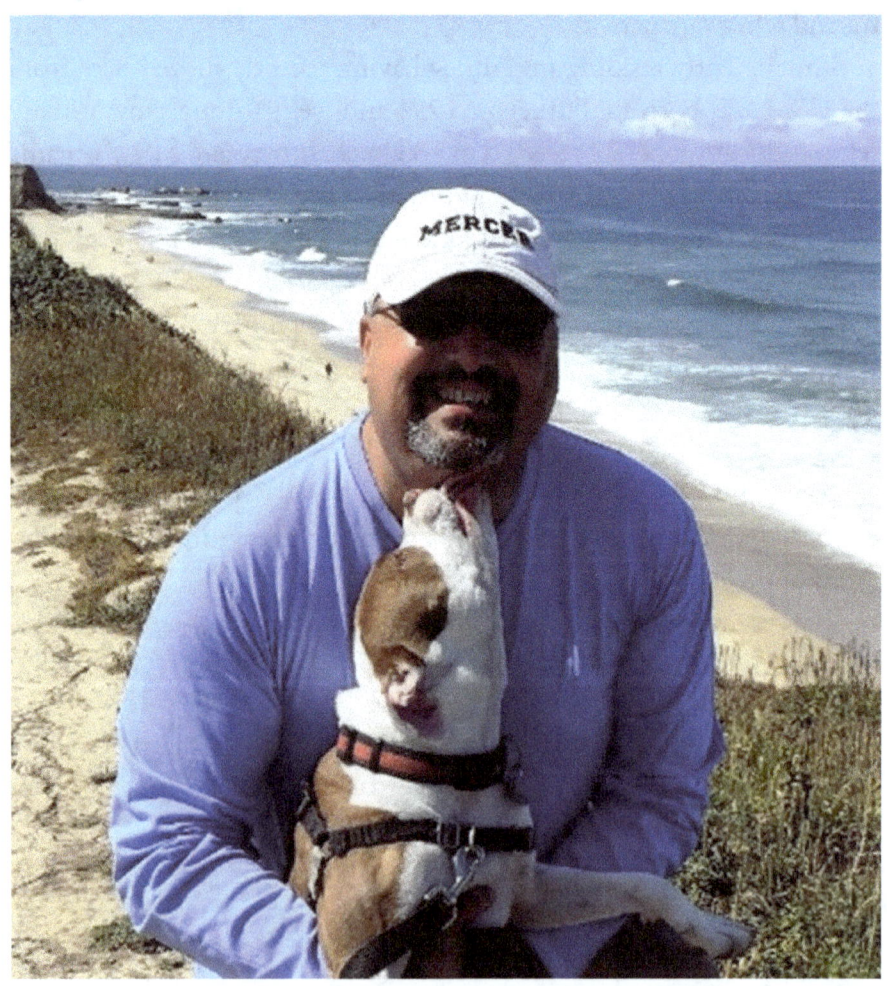

With Mica, a friend of a friend, in Half Moon Bay, California

# CHAPTER 1

# At 50 : The End! – or the Beginning

*San Diego, California, September 2005*

When I left home to go to my office, I had already told my wife that I might be back early that morning as I suspected I was going to be laid off.

I was living in San Diego with the rest of my family of four—my two children and their mom—and our Labrador retriever. My wife, Zeynep, and I had been married for twenty-three years and had explored the idea of divorcing twelve years earlier because of irreconcilable differences. Having seen how miserable the kids were during the separation, however, we decided to come together and postpone the divorce until the kids were older and could handle the event better. We were getting close to this milestone, as our son, Kurt, was now eighteen and our daughter, Sibel, was fifteen.

I had been recruited by Accelrys in 1996 as a senior product manager, and over the next nine years was promoted to director, senior director, and finally executive director, with increasing responsibilities and authority at each advancement. At Accelrys, we provided computational chemistry software tools for chemical companies, and specifically supplied pharmaceutical and biotechnological companies with computer-aided drug design tools (CADD). The business was crowded and competitive, with insufficient money available to support all the players in this market. As a result, an inevitable shakeout started slowly but lasted for over a decade with a subsequent consolidation of companies through a series of mergers and acquisitions. Having acquired several companies early in this shakeout, Accelrys became one of the larger players in the market. I ended up having to decide the fate of numerous competing products from companies that we acquired; which ones would remain active and continue to be supported, which ones would be assimilated into the existing platforms, and which ones would be phased out. As such, my job became more and more stressful. The years of mergers and acquisitions, also saw successive changes in upper management. During the nine years leading up to 2005, I reported to several managers and had good relationships with all of them except for the last one.

I first suspected I was going to be laid off the previous week while I was on a routine week-long business trip to the United Kingdom with the cheminformatics group there. Cheminformatics involves chemical information management systems based specifically on chemical structures. They are similar to typical database management systems (DBMS) that are widely used to manage pretty much everything from corporate accounting and personnel data to schools' student records.

Cheminformatics DBMSs, however, take as their organizing base the molecular compounds' chemical structures, the arrangement of individual atoms in the molecule. This allows the users of these DBMS to search for chemical features and structural aspects of compounds in the database. This is essential for certain industries; in fact, pharmaceutical companies consider their proprietary chemicals to be their "crown jewels." It's the chemical structure that gives these jewels their inherent value, and it's the cheminformatics systems that let the companies mine these jewels.

Beginning several decades ago when cheminformatics systems became available, searching for chemicals in an organization's database quickly became an important research tool for designing new compounds or drugs. Scientists used queries specifying fragments of chemicals, or based on similarity to another chemical structure, to conduct these searches. Later, these system's capabilities moved from two dimensions (like the line drawings in chemistry books) to three dimensions (like the movable ball-and-stick models on a chemistry teacher's desk). Once three-dimensional (3D) information management systems became available, scientists could search a corporate database with 3D queries that involve spatial arrangement of abstract features (like acidic groups or lipophilic [fat-loving] groups). These 3D queries, called "pharmacophore models," became an indispensable research tool. Today almost all recent drugs are designed or discovered through these types of CADD tools.

During my trip to the Cambridge office, I received a voice message from my boss asking (actually, demanding) me to cancel the rest of my trip and return to the office in San Diego as soon as possible. He gave no further explanation. This was early September of 2005. I now had to find a replacement for the second leg of my trip to Dublin to give a presentation at a conference. I was thankful that one of my product managers was readily available to take my place.

I moved up my return flight back to San Diego. On my last night in Cambridge, I invited my associates for a dinner at my favorite Turkish eatery, Efes Restaurant. This dinner banquet had become a tradition whenever I had business in Cambridge. My colleagues and I would feast on around half a dozen hot and cold appetizers, each have a main course, and finish with some great dessert choices.

As we dined, we talked shop, this time speculating on the future possibilities for the cheminformatic business at Accelrys. This business had fallen out of favor with the new management who had come in to turn around the company's faltering business, a small part of which was cheminformatics.

We recognized that a flawed internal accounting system ended up making the chemistry business' sales look worse than they were. For example, when a big sale involved both biology and chemistry products, Accounting needed to figure out which product was the one that persuaded the client to go with our solutions. This was complicated by the tendency of the account representatives to package additional products into the sales to make the total amount higher (for which the salesperson earned commission). I much later learned that some of the account reps would credit the added biology products for the original sale because they were "good buddies" with the biology director. I was not "buddies" with any of the sales reps, so my team ended up getting credit for the sales of just our products, not the overall sale, even if the chemistry products drove the overall sale. We knew at the time that upper management perceived the chemistry part of the business to be contributing less than it was, even without the compounding "buddies" influence that we weren't yet aware of as we dined that night.

\* \* \*

If you had asked me in those days what would be the worst thing that could happen to me, I would have said "losing my job." We were a single-income family with a mortgage in Southern California and two kids, one of whom was just starting college and the other finishing high school. There were a lot of bills to pay, which made losing our only means of support seem dreadful. My wife, Zeynep, used to work while we were in the San Francisco Bay Area but decided to stay at home to take care of the kids when we moved to San Diego. I had appreciated the sacrifice she was making at that time, and the kids ended up being raised in a healthy and supportive environment. But now that the children were grown, we could have used some added income in these trying times. During the previous several months, I'd been warning Zeynep that I might not be able to survive at the company given its circumstances and that she should seriously consider looking for at least a part-time job to allow for a smooth transition in case I lost my job. She ignored these warnings.

By that time, my relationship with Zeynep had only worsened since the dysfunction that led to our first attempt at separation twelve years earlier. With stress at work and stress at home, I felt like I had nowhere to go and no one to talk to. I felt alone, carrying a load of responsibilities with no hope for relief or support.

\* \* \*

During that last dinner in Cambridge, we were playing a game of sorts, brainstorming scenarios for the future of this cheminformatics business, all of which involved some type of a parting from the main company, either through a spinoff or a sale. Mishi was my counterpart in Cambridge responsible for the development of the cheminformatics systems. Our excellent relationship meant an effective workflow for product planning, management, and development. The processes we developed became a benchmark at Accelrys for successful team management of a complex business.

Given that relationship, Mishi shared with me that he, some people on his development team, and even some of my product managers in the Cambridge office would all be happy to put down their own money to spin off the chemistry business because they believed that it could be much healthier under different management. Contrary to the new Accelrys management, they appreciated the higher value of this business.

The option I liked best was to find an external buyer—and I already had a company in my mind for that: Symyx Technologies. At that time, Symyx was headed by Steven Goldby, who had been the chief executive officer (CEO) of my previous and much-loved employer Molecular Design Limited (MDL), where I had worked for many years. I respected him. Symyx was specialized in informatics and automation products. I felt they would appreciate how our cheminformatics solutions for life sciences complemented Symyx' own cheminformatics solutions for materials science. But we had no authority to entertain such transactions, and we believed the new management would have ignored any such suggestions. The exercise was futile, merely casual fun among friends.

* * *

This was not the first time I had been summoned back to headquarters during a business trip in Europe. A summons five or six years earlier came after a series of private conference calls to give me a heads up of what to expect. I was to take over the product responsibility of this very cheminformatics business in Cambridge, UK, after Accelrys had acquired it a year earlier.

With the cheminformatics business added to the chemistry business that I already oversaw in San Diego, I would become responsible for all the chemistry products in the company and would be promoted to executive director from senior director. I was elated. This looked like a wonderful promotion.

There was no such position at Accelrys at that time; management created this executive director position specifically for me. I felt flattered to become the highest ranked director in the company. Thinking about this promotion more deeply as I faced my second unexpected summons, however, I realized this may have been me hitting my glass ceiling. It seemed like they did not want to promote me to a vice president position. I was not in the inner circle; I kept to myself. And this was by choice. I didn't want to participate in a superficial environment where it seemed everyone was angling for power and benefits. I was a scientist, expecting my performance to carry me up the corporate ladder. My focus had always been the science of our business, not company politics. So I had not socialized with the people in management. I did not attend their BBQ parties, did not join their golf outings, did not hang out with them during business trips. Doing so was not in my nature, and I saw no reason to pretend it was simply to play politics.

Initially, I was hesitant to take the executive director offer, since I thought this would be too much work and responsibility for me at a time when I was already feeling overwhelmed. After several hours of meetings, where many of my concerns were addressed, I did accept the promotion, still with some hesitancy though. That had been about five years before this latest summons.

This time, however, there were no private meetings or heads-ups before my summoning. So, I expected unwelcome news; for sure it would not involve a promotion. In the past several months, I had increasingly grown at odds with the new management. The industry shakeout continued. The company was failing, and the newly formed management consisted of people who considered themselves turn-around specialists. I perceived their focus to be on preparing the company for sale rather than fixing its problems to prepare for its long-term success.

The leadership's initial focus seemed to be on making the numbers look good. They had a checklist to implement. This may have worked fine for their earlier operations, but it wasn't quite applicable to our different business model. For example, one would expect that management would carefully analyze how the company operated, what worked and what did not, and identify critical personnel. None of this was happening. In fact, the new management was unaware they were already losing critical employees. If they had been truly interested in turning the company around, they would have identified these people and made the necessary assurances to keep them on board. In my opinion, they were more interested in making a quick sale, collecting their commissions, and moving on. They would simply use the tactics they used at prior companies as templates and implement them at Accelrys. Of course, one of the first things they considered was reducing headcount. By then, most of the people I liked and trusted had already left the company and found opportunities elsewhere. I was one of the few people from my generation who remained despite the work stress. As I accepted more and more responsibility, I had to become increasingly efficient. But as I managed to complete my increased workload, even more came my way. My already long workdays were no longer adequate to succeed. I remember waking up in the middle of the night, covered with sweat, mentally screaming repeatedly "I have to get out of this place! I have to get out of this place!"

Why hadn't I considered leaving the company? Because I was deluded that things would get better, and I aspired to one day become the chief scientific officer of the company. When I had started at Accelrys about ten years earlier, it branded itself as having a high percentage of employees with PhDs. No longer. At first, like other respected science-based companies, Accelerys attracted employees largely from the highest level of scientific academia, where collaborating and working together is the norm and collegiality is common practice—not infighting, backbiting, sucking up, and internal competition. In retrospect, the shift in the company culture from science and technology to marketing and sales was apparent, yet I had failed to see this shift and was living in denial.

With these thoughts in mind, I started my drive to work that fateful morning to meet with my boss, whose name, let's say, was Brian. He was tall, brunette, and seemed to spend a lot of time in the gym as he was impressively built. With his thick mustache, he reminded me of a typical Californian surfer dude rather than a vice president of a high-tech company.

The meeting with Brian was at 7:30 a.m., first thing in the morning. I went directly to his office. His large, L-shaped corner office boasted outside walls made of glass, offering outstanding views on two sides. When we were moving to this new building about a year earlier, Human Resources (HR) was struggling with a shortage of offices. They originally assigned to me, the most senior member of his team, the large, rectangular office right next to Brian's. It also had good views and was large enough to put in a separate meeting area with a large white board and a table with four chairs. The only problem was that it was right next to Brian's office.

As I already hinted, I did not like Brian much and really did not want to be nearby where we would bump into each other frequently and would have to socialize. So, I proposed a win-win solution of moving to a smaller office further down the corridor and to partition the large office originally assigned to me into two smaller offices for two of my product managers. The company would get an extra office, two of my product managers would get window offices, and I would be far away from Brian. But this distance may have exacerbated my deteriorating relationship with him.

The meeting on this day was short and to the point: I was being laid off. I was to go to HR to receive my paperwork and make an appointment to come back another day to retrieve my personal items. I was to leave the building at once.

* * *

Brian was clueless as to the science and technology of our business. His focus was on company politics. He did not spend any time trying to understand the science behind the products or getting to know the people on his team and what they did. In short, he was always nurturing those above, never those below.

A few months earlier, my group was celebrating publishing an important book to which we had contributed a chapter. Brian showed up and seemed impressed that we had been invited to contribute and asked, "How come?" I explained to him that the editor of the book was a friend of mine who had contributed to a book I had edited on pharmacophore modeling, and he then asked me to return the favor. Brian was surprised and asked, "You have a book?" He had not even bothered to look at our files.

Brian, for his part, perceived a lack of respect from his direct reports. One day, for instance, a product manager who had reported to me for several years but was then directly reporting to Brian came to me for advice when Brian was out of town. He had decided to leave Accelrys for another opportunity. Brian was in Japan, and the product manager was scheduled to join him there in the next few days but did not want to. I suggested he go to Japan, do his last bit of work, and take the time with Brian to talk about his plans. He did not take my advice but canceled his scheduled trip to Japan and submitted his resignation to HR. When Brian returned from Japan, he was furious at me because his report decided to talk with me instead of him. The fact that some of his people were seeking my counsel seemed to threaten him. When he received the directive to reduce headcount, it may have been a handy opportunity to get rid of me.

When I showed up at HR after my meeting with Brian, the HR manager had my paperwork ready for me. She wore a guilty expression, probably because I had been with the company for nearly ten years with an outstanding performance record and was the type of a person HR usually worked to keep on board. The paperwork was straightforward. It offered a modest package, one not available for voluntary resignations. There was one catch: I would have to sign a document agreeing to forego any legal action around my termination.

It was with this choice in my mind that I stepped out of my car after the short return trip home. I had such an exceptional performance record at the company that I should be able to take legal action for wrongful termination. I could fight to take my job back. But I did not relish the thought of going back to a job that had become so stressful, where neither the work nor the company provided a happy place any longer.

I remembered my start at Accelrys about a decade earlier. When I left MDL for Accelrys, I enjoyed going-away luncheons, accolades, appreciations of past performance, and heartfelt good-byes. My last boss at MDL took several days to debrief me before my departure. He wanted to learn my knowledge and perspective about the market directions, new prospects, the competition, and scientific developments in the field. He even asked me to postpone my start with Accelrys for two days because he was not done debriefing me. A year later when I was talking to the vice president of HR at Accelrys, she said "When I saw the email from your boss at MDL a day before your start date here with a subject line 'Osman Güner,' I was so worried that I called in the CEO before opening it." She thought MDL was going to pull the plug on my hire for competitive reasons. When she and the CEO finally read the email, they were relieved to see that all MDL was asking for was two more days to complete my debriefing.

This time, there was no debriefing. After nearly ten years at Accelrys, I had so much more knowledge about the very crowded, competitive market with detailed and relevant information about how to beat the competition. Brian did not want to know any of that. He just wanted me out of his way as soon as possible. There were no going away parties, no accolades for the years of service, nothing. That was how Accelrys sent me off, almost like a criminal.

And that was it. I thought about all the time that I could have spent with my children instead. After giving ten years of my life to this place, helping it grow, bringing on new talent, and lending all my accumulated industry expertise, I was finished.

My feelings about this dramatic change in my life surprised me. I didn't feel angry. I didn't rage. I didn't want to sue the company for wrongful termination. Instead, I felt embarrassed, ashamed. I felt like a failure. I had been respected as a beacon of success up to that point. What would all my professional associates think of me, now that I was laid off?

I decided not to contest the termination but to take the package and use the time it bought me to figure out what happy work I wanted to do in the future. From this point on, I would only do work I enjoyed.

I was particularly interested in carrying out drug design myself. After guiding so many scientists on how to use the technology over many years, I wanted to do what I had been preaching all this time. That meant either working for a pharmaceutical or biotechnology company involved in CADD or providing contract research for them.

\* \* \*

When I looked in the mirror the next morning to shave, I saw a tired, unhappy face. I was almost fifty years old. I was in a dysfunctional marriage with two great kids, a lovely house that I had mostly paid for but that felt like it didn't belong to me, and a Mustang convertible I loved to drive. Kurt had just started at Gonzaga University, which had a very strong basketball program. Sibel, was a junior in high school and the co-captain of the speech and debate team. She was just starting to consider college options and had already decided on the East Coast. We couldn't persuade her to pick a university in California where we would pay in-state tuition. We'd helped her to develop wings, and now she wanted to fly off.

My kids were both bright, but the similarities ended there. While Kurt envisioned getting married, putting down roots, and raising a family, Sibel wanted to travel the world and experience different cultures.

As for myself, only months before my fiftieth birthday, I was unemployed—for the first time in my adult life.

\* \* \*

Postscript:

- Accelrys let Brian go a year or so after my departure
- 2007 – Symyx acquired MDL
- 2010 – Accelrys merged with Symyx

- 2014 – Dassault Systèmes acquired the combined company, which still exists today

# CHAPTER 2

# Before 50 ; Career Beginnings

## *Ankara, Turkey, 1956-1979*

When I was a kid growing up in Turkey, around age seven, I remember attending a science fair. A large laptop-sized machine on display (considered a primitive calculator today) performed only four types of calculations: addition, subtraction, multiplication, and division. Very gently, I pushed down the button labeled "2". Then I pushed down "+", then "2" again; and holding my breath, I slowly pushed down "=". The "4" I saw displayed was the most amazing thing I had ever seen. I thought to myself, "When I grow up, I hope I will be wealthy enough to afford one of these machines."

I don't remember how I learned to read. No one had taught me. I think I connected sounds with letters of the alphabet. Turkish is a phonetic language, so the letters always sound the same (unlike in English, for example, where the sound of "oo" can vary, as in book versus door). So I must have recognized the patterns of sounds for common street signs. By the time I started elementary school and acquired my first schoolbooks, I could read and comprehend. I was surprised that none of the other students could read.

I grew up in a traditional middle-class family in Ankara. My father worked as the general manager of the Turkish Historical Society, my mother was a home maker, and I had an older sister. My childhood wasn't especially happy. My parents argued a lot, and hearing their shouting matches from my distant room, I felt miserable. Yet a few minutes later, they continued with life as if nothing happened while I was still shaking in my room. This was their modus operandi for communicating with each other, never realizing the effect of their loud arguments on their children.

My authoritarian parents always expected us to do what we were told; my self-esteem suffered. My mother, the home maker, took care of us while my father, the bread winner, kept his distance. Mom cooked and made sure we always had nutritious food on the table and warm clothes in the winter. Despite my father's detachment, he did respect us and I enjoyed, occasionally, having somewhat adult conversations with him. My sister, Mine (pronounced me-neh), was four years older than I was, so we didn't play together. We had our own friends.

My father wrote a book entitled *Peynir Ekmek* (Cheese and Bread). It was a fictionalized story about his attempt to study and emigrate to the UK and his short time there trying to survive during the depression after World War II. This book may have planted the early seeds of my ideas for attending school overseas and perhaps even emigrating. The book received some acclaim. My father was depicted as a young new writer emerging from the ruins of war. It was a one-hit wonder, though; he didn't consider writing another novel.

During that time of depression in Turkey, the publisher was having a hard time paying royalties for the book's sales. He instead offered to pay by giving my father a copy of all the paperback books they had published. That's how I ended up having access to hundreds of books growing up, including the Turkish translation of all the classics. This was wonderful. I loved reading, and all these books let me experience different cultures around the world, sparking a life-long interest in global customs and traditions.

My father was not much of a risk taker. Starting from modest beginnings, he was acutely aware of the consequences of poverty and wouldn't take any chances while raising two kids. A judge friend of his wanted him to consider purchasing a condo unit in a building his son was constructing in Marmaris, a resort and vacation area on the Mediterranean Sea. My father was not interested because of the multi-year monthly mortgage commitment. But my mother pushed him to invest in two units: a corner unit at the end of an internal cul-de-sac, and a smaller unit right next to it. Before the deal closed, Mom coincidentally overheard my father talking on the phone with his judge friend. Apparently, the bill was too high for my father, and he was considering backing out. The judge was giving a last-minute warning as there were several prospects interested in investing. My mother immediately grabbed my father's arm and rushed to the judge's office. She was not able to get the second unit but was able to secure the end unit.

Our waterfront condo boasted 180-degree views of Marmaris Bay. From the left (i.e., east), you could see the city of Marmaris' walkway snake from about two miles away through beachfront all the way to our condo and continue west another four miles to a town called İçmeler. The coast resembled Malibu Beach in California, but with a closed bay that looked like a large lake instead of open ocean, and a walkway separating the buildings from the beach. During the summer, the many tourists from the full waterfront hotels and resorts jam-packed the beach with beach chairs and umbrellas. It was noisy, crowded, and hot. During the fall, however, at the season's end, the hotels closed, and the beach chairs and umbrellas disappeared, revealing Marmaris' natural beauty. (And the birds returned). From our condo, Marmaris Bay looked like a lake as interlacing mountain cliffs made the open end of the bay appear closed. My mother's intervention secured for us this lovely waterfront condo in Marmaris where I have spent all my remaining summers.

One of my father's passions was philately: stamp collecting. He exhibited in Europe, was the president of the Ankara Philatelic Association and took leadership roles in the Federation of European Philatelic Associations. He often said he was looking forward to his retirement when he could spend all of his time with his stamps. He also wrote two nonfiction books about stamps. Occasionally, he would take me to the weekly meeting at the Ankara Philatelic Association where I enjoyed being able to spend time with him. After a while, I came to be a recognized face, and people started to look at me as one of the possible future leaders of the philatelic society.

I was an enthusiastic Boy Scout in those days. So, when my father encouraged me to develop a thematic stamp collection, I decided on scouting as my theme. Many stamps featured the Boy Scouts, and I enjoyed organizing them in a way that complemented the written information about them. For example, if I found a stamp with a knot on it, I would display the stamp next to the actual knot. My father took my collection with him to one of the exhibitions in Europe, where it received a commendation, launching my career in philately.

My father wanted me to put together a new stamp collection about the life of Turkey's great modernizing hero, Kemal Atatürk. He thought this collection would win more awards even than the scouting effort. I was okay with that, initially. Once the work started, however, my father would frequently interfere and suggest changes and then practically take over. When we finished, I didn't feel like I owned it. As my father predicted, it ended up winning awards. However, I figured that if I were to continue with this hobby, I would always be in my father's shadow, and I didn't want that. So, I quit philately.

As a teen, I would read one magazine cover to cover. It was called "Bilim ve Teknik" (Science and Technology). I aspired early to be a scientist. But what sort of a scientist, I didn't yet know. I figured it out in my senior year of high school. At my school, mathematics, chemistry, physics, and biology were required classes. In our senior year, we could elect to take more advanced science courses. I took organic chemistry. Organic chemistry explores the chemistry of carbon-containing compounds, the fundamental components of all life forms. The depiction of organic chemical structures especially attracted me. It was like a code, and I was fascinated by simple code breaking at that time. I had even created a new alphabet, and a few of my friends and I would exchange coded letters using it and have fun deciphering them. My organic chemistry teacher, Vitali Meşulam, inspired us so much that I fell in love with organic chemistry, and I now knew my future: I was to become a chemist.

I wasn't a top student in high school. I settled for above average by studying just enough to get by. Rather, I focused on my hobbies. Scouting took a lot of my free time. I was also on the high school fencing team and in the school-band playing the tenor horn. When I left the band during high school, I realized that I was missing music and purchased a trumpet, which I played privately for many years. I dramatically changed this relaxed approach to high school during my senior year to get ready for the national university entrance exam.

Getting into a university in Turkey was extremely competitive those days, with spots available each year for only the top five to ten percent of all graduating seniors. This was before many private universities sprouted in Turkey in the years following. Worried about the low odds, I took prep classes in the evenings during my entire senior year. I didn't want to leave anything to chance.

My eyes were on one of the top universities, Middle East Technical University (METU). The application process for all Turkish universities included a nationwide exam (much like the Scholastic Aptitude Test in the US). Acceptance was based on a combination of exam results and a student's stated order of preference for a field. When I applied to METU, it required a separate entrance exam, so I needed to take two exams, one for METU and the second for the other Turkish universities. It didn't worry me that the classes at METU were taught in English.

I had started learning English in elementary school. In high school, I picked German as my required second foreign language. I felt comfortable with English, and only became aware of my heavy accent much later, when I traveled to the US. My German, though, never went beyond basic conversational level, and over the years I've forgotten what little I knew.

The METU exam preceded the national one. I thought I did okay. The list of admittees was to be published in the newspaper on a certain date. One morning my father, euphoric, woke me early, flourishing the newspaper. He had been so worried about the outcome that he arose ahead of the paper's arrival. My name was the fourth from the top for the chemistry department. Since I was able to get into my top choice for both the university and the field, I no longer needed to take the national exam. I was going to be a student at METU. This was important for me, a new world opening. I was happy.

While getting accepted was challenging, the cost of university education in Turkey was practically free. The tuition was low, but the books were a more significant expense, since the textbooks were imported for our education in English.

METU sat just outside the metropolitan area west of Ankara. Like many large college campuses, it was almost an independent small town, with academic buildings, labs, dorms, a little post office, and lots of places to buy snacks, including several cafeterias and a small market. It had a large library with rooms for group study and social club meetings. A bus system shuttled regularly to and from the city and throughout the campus. A gymnasium, a stadium, and other amenities for athletic events offered plenty of opportunities to stay fit. I joined the fencing team and continued to fence at the university facilities with barely a pause from my high school practice. Full-time students could spend their entire days on campus, attending class, enjoying meals, exercising, studying, socializing, and relaxing. I loved it.

Living on campus gave me time to develop personally. Twice a week, I ran a couple kilometers around the stadium track and then weight trained at the gym. Once a week I practiced fencing. Chess became my cerebral hobby at METU—the first of mind-challenging passions to eventually include competitive backgammon and competing at and teaching bridge and directing tournaments.

METU had a large contingent of chess players who gathered in one of the dozen or so cottages for social activities and clubs. The large cottage that housed the chess club magnetically pulled me towards it. I played there, read some books about chess, and started to improve. The active university club regularly organized tournaments, including games with departmental teams. Team tournaments were a lot of fun. My chemistry team held our own, trash-talking with players from different departments. By the time I finished my degree, I was respectable at chess (and decent at trash-talking).

* * *

Being shy and socially ill-at-ease, I had many acquaintances, but few true friends. Among them was my best friend, Hülya. Very bright, she wore her brown hair short and stood about five feet, five inches. We shared several classes in our first year at METU. We studied together and helped each other with freshman challenges.

Soon, we met others and formed a group of compatible students who would study and hang out together. During those years, METU was politically charged, and various political factions tried to recruit first-year students. Our group stuck together to dodge recruitment. We thought these groups were exploiting student goodwill and, in turn, were being exploited by outside forces. They were good, patriotic people, but we felt that competing Turkish political powers were using them. Our left-leaning crew supported our own political agenda without joining any of the factions' groups. Instead, we focused on our education.

Within a year, the turmoil eased when the right-wing factions were driven out. Bonded by our political hazing, our crew now spent more time simply socializing. Even though I still preferred solitude sometimes, it felt good to be part of a group: I belonged. As our friendships grew, during holidays we started to travel together and visit each other's homes (including occasionally my family's condo in Marmaris). Those good years of friendship set the bar high, and when I came to the US, I found that few people could clear it.

Our group became popular. As more people wanted to join us, we were becoming selective about whom to allow in. I liked one person, Kemal, who was friendly, charming, genuinely nice. At five feet, ten inches, he was athletically built and amiable. He also seemed to have a specific interest in Hülya and, importantly, was not threatened by our close friendship. One day Hülya and I went to watch Kemal play soccer in an amateur league. As right fullback, he was playing well until he collided with another player and went down. Hülya looked horrified. Apparently, the interest between them was mutual.

Meanwhile, my scouting activities continued full blast. Our group was part of an experimental group, the *Pioneer Scouts*. Our Turkish scout leaders created and refined this program as the next step, similar to the Eagle Scout concept in the US, to continue advanced scouting past high school and into college. To become a Pioneer Scout, you had to pass a general culture exam and complete a teaching or building project in one of the poor, rural areas in Turkey. Paired with another scout, you also had to survive a sixtyish kilometer walk through and one night camping in a thick forest. The program intrigued the World Scout Bureau, who was monitoring it. One of our leaders was the popular and friendly Yavuz Saral. Unfortunately, he was suffering from leukemia, which eventually took his life. Though expected, his death shocked most of us. He was the main pillar of the Pioneer Scout movement, and it phased out within the next few years after his passing.

It was during a gathering following Yavuz' funeral that I first met Zeynep. Slim and just five feet, three inches, she stood erect and proud, with brown hair and brown eyes. We exchanged only a few words, but I was intrigued. On our way back in the car with some of my scouting friends, I realized one of them fancied Zeynep. So, I decided to back off. Several months later, I checked with my friend and learned his interest had waned. I told him I would like to meet and get to know her. As it happened, we came together over scouting. An Ankara high school needed an assistant scout master, and my friends asked Zeynep if she would be interested in the position. She was, and when we met to discuss the process, I realized the attraction went both ways.

Zeynep was the only daughter of a retired three-star general, who was not yet ready to give up his daughter. The first time I met him at a small gathering at their home, I moved around the room shaking hands and introducing myself. When I came to him, he loosely shook my hand without looking me in the eye. I did not let his hand go until he raised his head and we made eye contact. He was shorter than my six feet, but his eyes were fierce and penetrating. I at once realized I would have to work hard to win him over. Aristocratic in her bearing, Zeynep's graceful mother seemed to like me, as I did her.

During our sophomore year, the spring semester of 1975, campus political tensions escalated. A dispute between the student organizations and the university administration resulted in students boycotting classes. I don't remember the reasons for the dispute, but we decided to support the boycott. Even though the classrooms were open, no one attended class. The student solidarity was impregnable. With this unexpected break, I decided to get a temporary job. One of my scout friends was working for a construction company, and I joined him there doing whatever needed to be done. The pay was dismal, but it kept me off the streets and put some money in my pocket.

The next semester the dispute was over, and the university reopened. We all received F's (which stayed permanently in our transcripts) for the courses we missed, and we had to repeat them. I decided to continue working at the construction company. I caught the bus to campus for my classes and, if there was a break between classes, caught the bus back to the city and to work. The hectic schedule was tough. Fueled by adrenaline, some days I would make the trip twice. I was too busy to keep up with my friends. I managed to finish the semester, barely passing with a C average. I realized that this was not sustainable and quit my job a day before the following semester began.

Back on campus full time, I didn't know what to do with the four hour break after my morning class. The hole in my schedule gave me a feeling of emptiness, after having rushed every minute for half a year.

Sitting on a bench contemplating, I saw Hülya and Kemal approach. They invited me for lunch. Seeing a good opportunity to catch up on group gossip, I agreed. They took me upstairs to the fancy faculty part of the cafeteria, complete with white tablecloths. This boded for a serious conversation. From their behavior, I suspected they were going steady. Kemal paid for our lunches, though Hülya usually paid for her own (in the cafeteria we paid the bill before we sat). And they were wearing matching beaded bracelets. Over lunch we caught up and shared what our friends had been doing during the break. We talked about everything except their relationship with each other. They seemed nervous to tell me their big news. Towards the end of the lunch, I couldn't wait any longer and asked them how long they had been together. They were relieved since they had been nervous about how I was going to take the news.

In Ankara those days, almost everyone lived in apartments or condominiums. Residence in private homes was rare. With Turkey's conservative culture, people did not live together when they were dating. A typical date involved going to pub or dinner or to private parties. Things got more formal when a couple got engaged. Still, even engaged couples generally would not sleep together until they got married. Of course, what went on behind closed doors is anybody's guess.

At lunch I learned not just that Hülya and Kemal were together but also that our group did not approve of this new more serious relationship and gave them a hard time. Eventually, the group broke up. Hülya and Kemal said they thought that if I had been around this wouldn't have happened, that I might have been able to bridge our friends' differences.

One day, I was driving with Hülya and Kemal to a friend's birthday party. Those were the early days of their relationship and Hülya's father instructed Kemal, rather firmly, that they shouldn't return after midnight. After the party on our way back, I suggested that we stop at a café for a drink and snacks. Kemal protested that we should go back home as he didn't want to miss his curfew and catch her father's fury. I said that I would take responsibility, and added, "When you were a kid running around in short pants, Hülya and I were best friends, and her father didn't see a need to enforce a curfew back then." The remark was a clear exaggeration, but he felt the insult.

Years later, when I was visiting them, married, and living in Istanbul, Hülya and I were trying to resolve a disagreement. We asked Kemal his opinion. He turned and said, "Are you asking my opinion?" and continued, "Was I not the one running around in short pants when you two knew everything there is to know in the universe?"

* * *

Full time on campus again, my life returned to normal except for our fractured group. I was still friendly with everyone, but our group was never whole again. Meanwhile the advanced classes were more demanding. With the first honeymoon years of college over, we had to focus more on our education. At one point, one of my professors told me that I could not get into graduate school with my current grade point average, so I went all-in during my last semester, getting all A's and managing to land the requisite grade point average for the graduate program. In Turkey, unlike in the US where one can directly apply for a PhD program, an MS is a prerequisite to a PhD.

My relationship with Zeynep was becoming more serious during our last two years in college. We continued to work on the scouting projects, went on picnics, and hung out. Zeynep was witty. Every now and then, she would make a funny comment that cracked me up during some of our serious conversations. We were fond of each other. And now Zeynep's father looked me in the eye when he firmly shook my hand.

By the end of our junior year, in the spring of 1978, we were engaged. Zeynep's family hosted our engagement party. They were cordial to my family from Istanbul and were almost perfect hosts. Zeynep and her family were now introducing me as her fiancé to some of their family friends. I felt they had finally accepted me.

Meanwhile, I saw signs of potential relationship problems. Zeynep was keeping a journal, and when she showed me what she had written about a particular event, I noticed that her perception about what had happened was different from mine. At the time, I just passed this off as a difference of opinion.

* * *

During the summer after graduation, the remaining members of our group spent part of our vacation together in Marmaris at our family's condominium. Now an intern at a military construction company, Zeynep couldn't join us. She was about to finish her degree in civil engineering at another university. Kemal was there with the group the whole time, while Hülya came later when all the rest of the gang were starting to leave. The three of us were the last ones there. Hülya and

Kemal were going to leave the next day, and I would spend an extra day cleaning up.

But tension filled the air. I found Hülya sitting in a lounge chair on the balcony looking miserable. She stared over the rail at the sea, the beach. Kemal was down there on the walkway also looking miserable.

"Hülya," I asked, concerned. "What's going on between you and Kemal? Why aren't you talking?"

"He's being very stubborn!" she said, some anger in her voice. "He doesn't understand why I need to live in Istanbul and build a career there."

Hülya had decided to live near her mother and family in Istanbul, with its abundance of job opportunities. The alternative was Ankara, where most of Kemal's family lived, and where we had all studied at METU. Kemal seemed to have an issue with her decision. I asked, "did you consult your boyfriend before making the decision?" She had not. I figured she was so focused on her own career that she hadn't thought about Kemal's needs, assuming he would simply go along with her decision. So, I did what any good friend would do: I bestowed my "wisdom" upon her. I said, "If you had done this to me, I would've left, yet Kemal is still here!" I also suggested that people who are planning to spend the rest of their lives together should make such critical decisions together. She was upset at first. How could I possibly take Kemal's side while being her best friend who was supposed to support her? But I could see that she was thoughtful and considering the situation.

Next, I went down to Kemal who was still sulking around the walkway. I explained how critical Hülya's career was to her, that the opportunities were much better in Istanbul, and that he should cut her some slack. Kemal also lashed out at me saying that of course I would take her side.

That night, an eerie silence engulfed our dinner. They were not talking, and both hated me for taking each other's side. While upset with me, they also started to consider each other's perspective. Later that night, when I was trying to sleep, I could hear them whispering together on the balcony. They were talking—mission accomplished! The next morning, I sent them off.

Much later, I learned the real reason of the conflict. Their relationship was getting serious and Hülya feared getting married before establishing her career. Despite landing a job at the biology department at METU, she decided to run to Istanbul to avoid having to make this important relationship decision in a rush. She had informed Kemal of her flight while they were visiting me in Marmaris. Kemal was also hesitant to commit to marriage at that time but was upset about Hülya's independent move.

Following a short separation, realizing that he was desperately missing her, Kemal went to Istanbul to woo Hülya and her parents. He charmed each member of Hülya's family and won them over one-by-one. The two eventually realized they could not live apart anymore and decided to marry about nine months after their confrontation in Marmaris.

They decided on an Ankara wedding (even though they were going to live in Istanbul) so that all their friends from the university could attend. Unfortunately, I missed it because my cousin Rengin was getting married in Istanbul the same day. Hülya and Kemal today remain happily married after more than forty years. Whenever I go to Istanbul, I stay with them instead of with my own relatives.

During my years living and working in the US, they came to visit me a couple times, and I in turn visited them a couple times in Turkey. Every four or five years or so we meet somewhere in the world and at once take up the conversations we left off five years earlier, as if no time has passed.

\* \* \*

The neighbor across from Zeynep's apartment was a teacher at the Ankara Conservatory. She said one of her friends who had a good pair of seats at the Symphony Hall was going to be in Canada for a year. Not wanting to lose their premium season tickets for the Presidential Symphony Orchestra, one of the top orchestras in Turkey, they asked if we would be interested in taking their seats that year. Both Zeynep and I like classical music, so we jumped at the opportunity. For that season, every Saturday we enjoyed the concerts from amazing seats, fifth row, center, at the Symphony Hall. When the program included a favorite piece, like Mendelson's violin concerto, we would also go to the rehearsals during the week before the performance on Saturday. Those were happy days when we enjoyed our favorite activities together.

* * *

During our junior and senior years of college, we could take elective courses. Most people took relatively easy and fun courses like photography and cooking. The elective courses I took were microbiology, radiation biology, and biochemistry. At my graduation, I had enough credits to pursue my master's degree in either chemistry or biology.

After getting my BS in chemistry, I took a semester off to figure out my next move. I knew I was going to enter a master's program but in biology or chemistry. During the semester break following graduation, Professor Okan Tarhan hired me to work for a few months on one of his funded projects. Because he was also the assistant president of METU, he was in the administrative building rather than the chemistry building where his lab was. My project involved natural product synthesis, and I would frequently gather my lab notebook and printouts from spectroscopic analyses and trudge over to the top floor of the administrative building, about a quarter mile away, for his feedback and guidance.

Emboldened by this work, I decided on a master's in organic chemistry. Professor Tarhan's project ended up being a good warm up for my master's program.

# CHAPTER 3

# MS at METU

*Ankara, Turkey, 1979-1981*

I was the first graduate student of a new Assistant Professor of Chemistry, Lemi Türker, for my MS study at Middle East Technical University (METU). (In most graduate programs, candidates are assigned to a professor who mentors them and helps direct their thesis.) Dr. Türker was short with metal rim glasses that seemed to heighten his intelligence. He received his doctorate at the University of East Anglia, England under a well-known scientist, Dr. Alan Katritzky.

Dr. Türker had diverse interests; for example, I later learned he was consulting for the National Theater Association on special effects (like pouring liquid nitrogen on stage to create instant fog) as a favor to a friend. He was also an artist. When I visited his home once to deliver a folder, I noticed that his walls were covered with hieroglyphic art he had drawn. His multidimensional curiosity and skills spanned science and the arts.

My master's work built upon his doctoral work. Its narrow focus on 1,3-dipolar cycloaddition reactions taught me valuable organic chemistry techniques. Cycloaddition reactions combine two chemical fragments to form a cyclic structure, like the classic hexagon shape with which even non-chemists may be familiar. When the initial fragments, the "reactants," have chemical components attached to them, called "substituents," the reaction produces multiple "isomers," meaning molecules with the same atoms, but with a different arrangement of those atoms or a different three-dimensional shape. The substituents may attach in different places on the resulting ring (forming "regioisomers") or position themselves either above or below the plane of the cyclic structure (forming "stereoisomers"). 1,3-dipolar cycloaddition reactions involve atoms other than carbon (called "heteroatoms"), like nitrogen or oxygen. The resultant ring structures are thus "heterocyclic" compounds, with atoms other than carbon included in the ring of the cyclic structure.[1]

Heterocyclic compounds are common in natural chemicals. As such, these reactions are useful to synthesize compounds in the lab that mimic natural compounds.

My supervisor was meticulous with lab procedures. We used advanced esoteric procedures like double-resonance nuclear magnetic resonance (NMR) imaging, preparative thin layer chromatography (TLC), and numerous "hacks" to synthesize organic chemicals.

Nuclear magnetic resonance provides information to identify chemicals. If you want to synthesize a new chemical, NMR is one of the most important spectroscopic techniques (i.e., a technique that measures the reflection of light and other electromagnetic radiation) to help validate the chemical's structure. This technique is familiar to patients under a different name. In medicine it is called *magnetic* resonance imaging (MRI) to circumvent people's fear of the word "nuclear." So, if you have undergone an MRI procedure, you were actually inside an NMR instrument (a rose by any other name…) that was using magnetic waves to look closely at parts of your body rather than at parts of a chemical compound.

Double resonance experimentation in NMR is an advanced technique to simplify the signals from waves bouncing off neighboring carbon atoms in a compound. The number of hydrogen atoms attached to neighboring carbon atoms dictates the complexity of the signal. So the complex data generated, simplified with this advanced technique, helps give a clearer picture of the arrangement of these molecular attachments.

Following my first cycloaddition reaction experiment, Dr. Türker was running the NMR on my sample as he taught me how to conduct the double resonance procedure. When he irradiated an area with especially complex signals, to his surprise the signals simplified to reveal that my reaction had produced the desired outcome. It was exactly the signal resolution (akin to a fingerprint) he was looking for, but apparently was not expecting, from my very first try. I suspect my work with Dr. Tarhan's project prior to the start of my master's helped me to develop some skills useful in synthesis. Dr. Türker's respect for me seemed to increase after this experiment.

I enjoyed and learned much from my collaboration with Dr. Türker. But eventually our relationship started to sour. Dr. Türker's relentless insistence on asserting control over me conflicted with my free spirit. (I had quit philately since I couldn't quit my dad, but I had no intention of quitting organic chemistry!) I felt he was learning how to interact with students by experimenting with me, his first graduate student. Soon after, a new graduate student lessened the pressure on me. I still did good work, but I tried to minimize facetime with my supervisor as much as possible.

I'm not sure why I had trouble submitting to authority. If I had an idea, I would stubbornly pursue it, resisting any modifications my supervisor suggested. He was naturally frustrated at my resistance, and we started to clash. I was not a good student who followed instructions, and this annoyed him.

During the first year of my master's, two research fellowship positions, akin to research professorships, opened in the department. Those selected would receive a lucrative salary and benefits at a level only slightly below a tenure-track assistant professor. It was an ideal steppingstone toward an academic career in Turkey. I was not yet sure if I wanted to pursue an academic career, but I wanted the option in case I did.

The requirements were stiff including a difficult written and a one-on-one oral exam. The selection committee was especially thorough since the two winners would likely be future fellow professors. A dozen applicants competed including me and the other graduate student from our group. Professor Türker spent a lot of time teaching and training the other graduate student for this exam.

Zeynep and her mother were supportive, and they kept saying that I would surely get one of the spots. Rather than make me feel supported, this angered me. Did they not realize how long the odds were? I was competing against the smartest eleven people in one of the top universities in the Middle East. I was terrified, haunted by my low self-esteem. I kept questioning why I had even tried; what was I thinking?

Following the written exam, the selection committee spent an entire day interviewing the candidates. One by one they invited us in. Each time, an hour later a devastated and disheveled candidate visibly sweating and sometimes also in tears left the room and the next victim was invited in. My supervisor's protégé was among the first five called in. As soon as he was finished, he and Dr. Türker retreated to his office to go over the questions. The rest of us were waiting nervously to be called in and some looked ready to collapse. I was the tenth person in line. Once the selection committee was done torturing the ninth candidate, they told the last three of us that they were calling it a day and would continue the interviews the next day.

The next morning, I was the first interviewee. After waiting around nervously the day before and watching the post-exam condition of each interviewee, I was dazed. When I entered the room, I was surprised to find that the panelists were cordial and seemed to deliberately try to get me to relax. I was expecting to see them as monsters ready to tear me apart. They had plenty of tough questions and some trick ones as well. I did my best with the tough ones and narrowly avoided at least one trick question. They seemed to be playing with me and having fun with each other, and I also enjoyed the game. I wondered why the people the previous day had been so exasperated. I felt good about the whole experience. Overall, I thought I did okay. The last two candidates were interviewed, and we would know the two winners the next day.

To my surprise, I received one of the fellowships. For a few days, I was numb. The realization had not quite sunk in. Yet when Dr. Türker congratulated me, he didn't seem surprised, as if he had always expected me to win. My parents' response to this fellowship was like indifference. They had said, of course, that they had no doubt I would get the fellowship. If only I could be so confident in my own capabilities.

It took three months to sort out the bureaucracy, and my first three-months' salary arrived all at once in a large paper bag—in cash. Most of the faculty had their salaries direct deposited into their bank accounts, but I didn't even have a bank account yet. I had never seen so much money before. I ended up buying lavish gifts for all my family members, my fiancé, and some close friends too.

My new job offered perks beyond the salary and respect that comes with being considered a faculty member. A new faculty tag for my car let me park at more convenient reserved spots around campus. The university owned a lake away from the campus. Zeynep and I would frequently go to there, hanging out. Even there, I could park in a premium spot.

* * *

The chemistry faculty volleyball team was looking for a player to add to their team and asked if I would join them. I had played a lot of street volleyball when I was growing up and loved it. I could have fun and meet faculty beyond the realm of chemistry.

So, I showed up for a game. They were looking for a setter, the player who stays close to the net and is fed the ball to set for the hitter, who sends it over the net. I would've been better as a hitter, but I decided I could do the job. I did my job, and the rest of the team was ecstatic. Finally, they had found a specialist player to complement the team. I became aware that other faculty watching the game were cheering for number 7. It took me a while to figure out that they were cheering for me. I had put on a fencing practice shirt, red with a large university logo on the front and number 7 on the back. I enjoyed playing, and it gave me something to talk about with the other faculty in passing.

After a few games, it almost felt like I was popular. Popular? Can you imagine a shy, solitary guy like me being popular?

Meanwhile, I continued playing chess. My best result in Turkey was when I finished with a five-way tie fifth-ninth in the Ankara Championship in 1980. I was happy with this result, and, when people asked, I would proudly say I was the ninth-ranked player, that year, in Ankara. This was good enough for me as Ankara boasted a population of close to a million people at that time. One day one of my chess player friends heard this and asked why I was telling people that I was ninth in Ankara? I should be saying I was fifth. Obviously, all the other players I tied with must have been better than me. That was my low self-esteem at work again, something that would continue to dog me, even long after I had proven myself.

Eventually during my studies, I needed to figure out my next step. I had been thinking about going overseas for my doctorate since reading my father's novel as a child. I decided that getting a PhD in the US (as opposed to Europe) would help me with better career choices in Turkey, whether I stayed in academia or moved to industry. Most of the companies hiring preferred American PhDs—don't ask me why. Regardless of where I went, I would be the first PhD in my family. I was happy that my father supported my plan enthusiastically.

Towards the end of my master's program, I started to apply to American graduate schools. One problem: I was worried about the F grades in my college transcript from the boycotted semester. Even though a footnote explained the situation, I didn't know how American universities, so far away, would interpret this anomaly. The transcript was one of the most important items in the application package.

I needed financial support, but with the F grades in my transcript, I didn't think I would qualify for the scholarships (like Fulbright) awarded to outstanding students. So I needed to secure financial support from the university as part of my application process. Most of the top colleges require the first year of classes completed before considering a candidate for financial support, and I couldn't afford to live in the US for an entire year despite my family providing us some startup money. So, I focused on a few universities where paid teaching assistantships were broadly available.

I didn't ask my supervisor for a recommendation letter. I was still acting stubborn and stupid in my relationship with him. Some other chemistry faculty members wrote one on my behalf, and I thought that would suffice. One day, Dr. Türker came to my office and handed me a dozen signed recommendation letters he had written for me, in open envelopes, and then he left. The letters were amazing: strong, supportive, beautifully written. Unfortunately, I didn't have a chance to use them since all my graduate school applications were already completed. Dr. Türker's gesture opened my eyes. Many years later, when I asked him why he did not help me to prepare for the exam even as he helped the other student, he told me that the other student desperately needed his help. We did part on friendly terms at the end of my master's program, and I still think of him as my first mentor who helped me to develop my strong and disciplined approach to scientific research.

After you complete your master's coursework and thesis and your professor approves the thesis, you face one last scrutiny: The oral defense of the thesis in front of a faculty committee. The committee ensures that the candidate knows the details of his or her work enough to defend it against other skeptical scientists. My thesis defense was straightforward, almost boring.

Still assistant president of the university at that time, Professor Okan Tarhan, was also on my committee. At one point, he mentioned a recent scientific paper related to the work I was doing, and I at once recited the full citation of the paper, with which I was intimately familiar. He turned back to the committee members and asked if they remembered any other candidate who could recite the full bibliography of any paper during their defense. With such support from the influential assistant president, the rest of my defense went smoothly. I received my MS degree in organic chemistry shortly thereafter towards the end of the Fall 1981 semester, and a few weeks later I headed for my mandatory military service.

* * *

Military service in Turkey was unavoidable. You could delay it with advanced schooling, but you couldn't eliminate it. One of the first things people ask during a job interview in Turkey is whether you had completed your military service (to assess if there would be an interruption in the candidate's employment later if the military service was not completed). If not, for example, you could only renew your passport for one year at a time. If I was to head overseas for my doctorate, I would need to visit the nearest Turkish consular office once a year to keep my passport up to date. Paying money to get out of the military service was not an option then. Later, people who were working overseas could pay a fee (about $10,000) and fulfill their military duty in one month—but such an expense would have been out of my reach anyway.

The assignment location was supposed to be random, but connections landed some in the nicer facilities near one of the major cities. Other folks would likely end up in smaller rural areas with poorer facilities. Zeynep insisted that I leverage my connection. Her father was a retired three-star general and still had tremendous influence in the military. But could I bring myself to ask for his help? By this time, you may already know the answer. I was still stubborn and stupid. In retrospect, if I had asked for his help, my relationship with him might have been better. I would perceive his help as submitting to his superiority, but life would have become easier for me. I've learned through this and other scenarios that I was terrible at asking for favors and even worse at accepting them.

With luck, I was able to complete my mandatory military service in merely four months. I took advantage of a temporary law change enacted to reduce the number of people eligible to serve as officers (i.e., people with advanced degrees). By agreeing to do the military service as a private, I could complete it in four months rather than in two years as an officer. Getting my military service out of the way before starting my doctorate was important. Otherwise, I might have to do it later when I would be busy trying to build a career.

I had sent my university applications during the last six months of my MS work and received several acceptance letters while serving in the military. I chose Virginia Commonwealth University (VCU) in Richmond, Virginia, partly because one of my professors in Turkey had done his PhD there, and his former supervisor, Professor Donald Shillady, was willing to help me get started. In addition, the department offered me a teaching assistantship from the get-go. In fact, they suggested that I consider coming to Richmond a few months earlier in May so that I could work during the summer as a teaching assistant before starting my doctorate in the fall of 1982.

This schedule worked out well for me. Zeynep and I were planning to get married in April. So, we could leave for the US a few weeks after the wedding.

The wedding was amazing. My parents booked a large space in a hotel in the downtown area for the reception. We went to the city registrar first for the official ritual and signatures. Only a few close relatives attended this part. Then all the guests dined at a lavish reception. Despite their financial constraints, I appreciated my parents' ability to put together this wedding. After the signatures and the traditional "I do's" we moved to the hotel.

Zeynep and I were resting in a room on the top floor of the hotel. Unbeknownst to us, we were supposed to wait to be called in, but no one mentioned this detail. So, after waiting and relaxing for a while, we decided to join the reception. We called the concierge, who let us know it was too early to show up there. But an escort promptly appeared to navigate us through the hotel. With our escort's lead, we slowly progressed through the labyrinth of a hotel. We were paraded through a large, busy dining area where applause welcomed us. A couple with a wedding gown and tux apparently was good promotion for the hotel, so we briefly became the focus of entertainment while we slowly made our way to the reception.

When we finally arrived, they were ready for us. Wedding music and more heartfelt applause accompanied us to our table. Almost all our relatives and close friends were there. Hülya had made the trip from Istanbul.

Following the reception, we nervously tied up loose ends for our voyage to the US—a first big trip to anywhere for both of us. We would have been lost without my parents' and sister's support in navigating all the hidden reefs and shoals of this major relocation. Zeynep's father kept anxiously asking about the process, which I repeatedly elaborated for him. First, we would go to Marmaris for our honeymoon, then fly to London. After an overnight stay there, we would jet to Washington, DC and then take a commuter flight to Richmond. Dr. Shillady would greet us there and take us to his home for a night before we'd move to our rented room near the university. Zeynep's mom apologized for the repeated questions from her husband and thanked me for being patient with him.

Zeynep and I had a relaxing week-long honeymoon in Marmaris. Since the season for tourism hadn't started then, it wasn't crowded and noisy. That fun week together provided a needed break from all the hassle.

We returned to Ankara to finalize our preparations. We had rented a room, in Richmond, in a small house right across from the chemistry department from the department chair who owned it as an investment property. With the arrangements completed, we started our trip to the US.

Heading to London, we settled into our seats on the Pan American jumbo jet. After a while, I noticed everybody talking English instead of Turkish. And suddenly, it hit me. This was it; no more parents or friends around; no more support. We were all alone on this big adventure. The resulting panic lasted only a few seconds, but it felt much longer. My anxiety eased as I started to mentally recite our itinerary (the way I had been reciting it to Zeynep's father). I started to relax. I could focus on all we would have to do as we started our new life.

In London, getting to our hotel near the Heathrow Airport with all our luggage was cumbersome. Our flight to the US was the next evening, so we went sightseeing in the morning around Piccadilly Circus. As we explored the area, an older gentleman passing by looked Zeynep up and down and touched his hat with a nod as he passed by. He seemed to appreciate her outfit. A dark blue conical strip fell diagonally across the front of her white dress and dramatically continued right across her matching shoes.

We headed back to the hotel to check into our flight to Washington, DC early (this was before smart phones) to get a jump on the processing wait involved with a full flight on a jumbo jet. Our little excursion of a metro ride to and from Piccadilly with a modest snack cost us more than a week's spending in Turkey, highlighting the cost-of-living differences between Turkey and UK. I assumed the US would be a similarly pricey.

# CHAPTER 4

# PhD at VCU

*Richmond, Virginia, 1982-1986*

I was glad we came to Richmond early since we were so green to life in the US. Like when we were doing all our grocery shopping at a 7-Eleven convenience store nearby, until the cashier, feeling sorry for us, pointed out the Safeway a block further where we could buy the same groceries for about half the price. Learning local ways during the summer gave us some confidence before I started my doctorate in the fall.

Zeynep and I were living in a single room but aspired to a better place once we learned our way around. Since our current residence was temporary, I rented a Post Office box so we wouldn't have to deal with an address change with each move. The mile walks every day to check our mail became part of my routine, later upgraded to a ride after we bought bikes. After about a year, we bought our first—cheap—car and getting around became easier. That heavily used car burned oil almost as fast as it consumed gasoline. The leaky head gasket repair would cost more than what we had paid for the car. But it served its purpose for about a year until we could afford to buy a better, newer used car.

Richmond is a beautiful city. But still, it took us Turks some time to adjust. The large urban campus of Virginia Commonwealth University (VCU) has facilities spread around the city—a jarring difference from Middle East Technical University's isolated and almost self-sufficient small town of a campus. Richmond was also expensive compared to Turkey. I started to worry about our finances. We'd been tapping into our savings, but we'd soon need additional income to make ends meet. I'd have to resolve that later, though. First order of business: getting familiar with the environment during the summer so I could focus on my studies without interruption in the fall.

The food was great. When I had my first Whopper® (which hadn't yet found its way to Turkey), I felt I was in heaven. The french fries in McDonalds were also great. This was before a wider awareness of healthy food—what to eat, what to avoid. But the best was the New York Delicatessen in the neighborhood. I could happily have all my meals there for the rest of my life.

At the start of the summer semester, I attended a meeting for the general chemistry labs in the amphitheater with about 60 students in the audience. The lead teaching assistant (TA) running the meeting pointed me out as one of the TAs for general chemistry. Towards the end of the session, he pointed to me and asked when my office hours would be. I didn't know what "office hours" meant, so I said I was not going to have office hours. I didn't even have an office yet. I was allocated a desk in a shared room with half a dozen other TAs. Lack of an office apparently did not matter. I was the only TA who did not have office hours that summer semester, perhaps a disappointment for the students in my section.

I did not have any examples of a prelab lecture and was too shy to ask for help, so I developed my own lectures. The summer semester completed quickly, and I enjoyed teaching it. I discovered that I had a heavy accent. The students seemed to enjoy my language challenges and took pleasure in correcting me. From them I learned to pronounce "thermometer" as one word, not as "thermo meter," and lots more. I encouraged them to correct my grammar, vocabulary, and pronunciation. As I taught them chemistry, they taught me English—a fair trade. The students patiently demonstrated the correct pronunciation of almost everything. Learning chemistry became less intimidating for them, seeing their instructor as a human being with his own limitations. Though Turkish chemistry students were more serious and hardworking, I found teaching American students to be more enjoyable. They were lively and seemed to understand that there is more to life than chemistry lab work.

My language difficulties quickly became apparent to more than just my students. Graduate students typically provided logistical support to guest lecturers giving seminars. For one such guest, I was tasked with loading his slides into the slide projector. At the end of the seminar, I returned the slides to him, and he thanked me for the help. I smiled at him, turned my back, and left. On my way out I heard him say something like, "Is it something I said?" He thought my lack of response meant I was angry about something he did. In reality, I didn't know what the proper response to "Thank you" was. Today, thirty years later, my two-year-old grandson, Ziya, knows when I say "Thank you" to respond with "You're welcome." I knew enough chemistry jargon to teach and debate it effectively for hours. As for verbal social lubrication, I lacked the fundamentals. I'm sure several times I've been considered rude because I couldn't come up with the simple, natural response to a question or comment. I suspect this is a common immigrant experience. Towards the end of the semester, all students from all chemistry sections gathered in the amphitheater for their final exam. This was the same large room where I announced at the beginning of the semester that I was not going to have office hours. The students spread out and nervously waited for the final exam to start.

Once it did, the students silently worked through the questions. One student asked for a clarification on a question. Since I had contributed it, I took it upon myself to respond thoroughly to all the students. I noticed that most of them looked confused and had no idea what I was talking about. I said, "If what I said doesn't make any sense to you, then you should not worry about it." That was the wrong thing to say, and I regretted it immediately. After the final ended, while students silently left the room, some of my students came over with some questions about the exam, but they all seemed to have done well. They were also saying their goodbyes, some asking whether I would be teaching this class or that, so that they could take another course with me.

After the semester's end, several students complained to the professor in charge of the general chemistry labs that those students in my section had learned more chemistry than the rest of them. They found the questions in the final based on the extra bits I had taught to be unfair.

At the beginning of the fall semester, when that professor stopped by, I prepared to be reprimanded for what I had said in the finals. He offered a more creative resolution. He asked if I would consider giving the prelab lectures not just to the students in my own section, but for all the sections in the fall semester. Still a bit naive, I said yes.

Around 300 students took general chemistry that semester, divided into fifteen lab sections of about twenty students each. Every morning, three sections that had lab scheduled that morning would gather for the one-hour prelab lecture and then disperse to the three general chemistry labs to run their experiments.

Monday mornings I would teach the prelab lecture for three sections and repeat the process for the next four days, giving the same lecture five times a week. I used transparencies that I had half-filled with a permanent black marker, and during the lecture I would complete the transparencies with an erasable black marker. At the end of the lecture, I would wipe the transparencies with a wet paper towel, and they would be ready for the next day's class. No personal computers and PowerPoint® presentations back then! The classes were a lot of work, but I enjoyed them, and they seemed to have helped me to establish myself in the department.

Based on how the students received Monday morning's lecture, I would improve the transparencies for Tuesday's class. Wednesday's class would receive my best lecture as I would have perfected the flow, transitions, and delivery. By Thursday, I would be tired and bored with the repetition, so I would lose some of my excitement and take shortcuts. By Friday, I would be so bored that this group would receive my shortest lecture, devoid of jokes and metaphors (colorful or otherwise), with just the basics. I didn't *want* to teach my late week classes this way, but my limited mental stamina demanded it.

I was curious to find out which group would perform the best in the finals. Naturally, I was expecting the Wednesday group who benefited from my "perfected" lecture to do the best. The actual results were surprising yet educational. Friday's group outperformed them all.

\* \* \*

Meanwhile, Zeynep and I signed up for an intramural volleyball team. We played in leagues every semester throughout our stay in Richmond, and during our last two years, we consistently won all the tournaments each semester. I also tried some other sports, like racquetball and Wallyball (volleyball played in a racquetball court) but didn't play as consistently. My volleyball stint left me with injuries, including a dislocated knee, a deformed pinky, and a shoulder pain that I carried with me for many years into the future. But the fun, fitness and camaraderie were worth it.

\* \* \*

After I settled into teaching, I explored the different VCU faculty's areas of interest to find a fit for me among all the interesting research going on at VCU. I was looking for a specific opportunity. I conceptually already knew what I wanted to do.

Doing my master's program in Turkey, I had been exposed to computers, and I wanted them to be part of my doctoral work. The mainframe at METU was an IBM® 360. Today, an average cell phone is more powerful. Though they were cumbersome and slow back then, I liked interacting with computers. I wanted to use my training in organic chemistry and my experience with chemical synthesis and spectroscopic analyses in my doctorate, and I also wanted to move towards theoretical chemistry, which tries to understand and explain complex general rules of chemistry that are not as yet proven. So, I sought a doctoral project that would have both experimental and theoretical components.

The professor who helped me settle into Richmond, Dr. Donald Shillady, was a physical chemist with several projects in quantum theory, which seeks to describe physical properties of nature at the minute scale of atoms and subatomic particles. He was developing a new "basis set"—an advanced technique to understand how electronic waves function via algebraic equations. I was intrigued but did not want to commit myself only to theoretical work. (Eventually I did contribute to one of his projects as a side activity that resulted in a theoretical paper published in 1987)[2].

Dr. Shillady had wire-rimmed glasses and wavy brown hair with streaks of white. He also had a gentle personality that I thought boded well for working with him as he supervised the theoretical part of my research.

My master's thesis had involved 1,3-dipolar cycloaddition reactions. Could I find someone who could leverage that but in theoretical chemistry? One of the professors at VCU, Dr. Raphael Ottenbrite, a Canadian, had done some work with another type of cycloaddition reaction called Diels-Alder reactions. At over 50, he was tall, blond and was still playing full-court basketball once a week with younger faculty and students. I hoped to be as athletic when I reached that age. After some consideration, I decided to take on both Drs. Shillady and Ottenbrite as my PhD supervisors and the departmental heads approved.

I would experimentally identify the cyclic products of a series of Diels-Alder reactions, then experimentally determine the regio- and stereo-selectivity and the distribution of the products. I would then run *ab initio* quantum mechanical calculations for these compounds and use the calculated orbitals to predict the reaction outcome through frontier molecular orbital interactions using second-order perturbation calculations. Say *what*? (I *told* you I was good with chemical jargon.)

In simpler terms, I would do the experiments and analyze the distribution of the products—that is, evaluate what those resulting various chemical "pearl necklaces" (see footnote 1) looked like. Then I would do calculations to predict the outcome theoretically and compare the theoretical results with the actual results. If I could come up with a method of reliable theoretical predictions, organic chemists could use them to sift through possible reactions to eliminate those predicted not to produce the desired compounds before going through the complex and expensive synthesis work.

Physical chemistry is one of the harder branches of chemistry, especially for someone with math challenges. It applies the concepts of physics—such as energy, force, and time—to chemistry, providing chemical concepts such as thermodynamics, quantum chemistry, and chemical reaction kinetics. Organic chemistry is also challenging but more specialized in the synthesis of new chemicals containing carbon – the stuff of life.

Half of my doctorate work involved experimental organic chemistry and the other half theoretical physical chemistry. This unusual synthesis of approaches let me compare the experimental results with theoretical predictions. I would receive my PhD as a physical organic chemist. It would take extra work to fulfil the requirements for two different and challenging branches of chemistry, but I thought it would be worth the effort. Once my advisors approved the proposed doctorate project, I began the research work in the fall semester of 1983.

*  *  *

My parents visited us that preceding summer, after my father sent $1,000 to cover their expenses while with us. That allowed us a vacation we could otherwise not afford. We scheduled a road trip to Florida and spent a week visiting Walt Disney World, Epcot Center—and one of my father's philatelist friends in Boca Raton. He and his family took us to their local clubs and showed us around the area. I appreciated this vacation in the midst working hard at the university with my research and teaching and so was grateful to my father.

*  *  *

Computer technology continued to advance but was still, compared to today, in the Stone Age. We could access the mainframe through dumb terminals with no computing power of their own from our desks. Large mainframe computers sat in the middle of huge elevated cool rooms. Computer scientists fed in the software programs with a series of cards, with each punched card representing one line of the program's code. Typical mainframe computer rooms, among other accoutrements, had card reading and card writing devices, printers, and miles of spooled magnetic tape to provide the storage space for the programs and for memory.

Dumb terminal screens did have keyboards and once connected to the mainframe, allowed users to type commands directly to it without the need for punch cards. You could write your own program, save it to a file on the mainframe, and read that file directly into the computer, eliminating the need for punch cards. While you could access the computer through a terminal, you still had to understand the operating system the computer ran on. This was before the operating systems and their arcane languages were hidden behind user-friendly windows. VCU mainframes ran a UNIX® operating system.

I was excited to access the university mainframe, so I taught myself the UNIX operating system. Once you master working with a mainframe through dumb terminals, you can do the same sorts of things we do today with personal computers (PCs were not yet widely available), albeit through a few more clunky steps. Soon I became the designated go-to guy in the chemistry department for all things related to computers.

One morning, when I arrived on campus, I noticed one of the faculty members furiously pulling out memos from the departmental mailboxes. He was mumbling that he would catch and expel the person who did it. Apparently, someone pulled a practical joke, writing a nasty letter using his name, matching the format of a departmental memorandum, and distributing it to all mailboxes. I arrived too late to see it, so I did not know what all the fuss was about. However, not many people had the skills to use the then new computer technology to mimic the memo format and forge a letter so well. I was afraid I might be on top of the list of suspects, though it would be hard to imagine me writing the letter with my broken English. At any rate, I decided to find out who had done it just in case I became a suspect.

It took me merely twenty minutes to find the culprit, thanks to my new-found facility with the UNIX operating system. I got the list of everybody who had accessed the mainframe the previous evening and found only one person from the chemistry department. He had been on the system between midnight and one a.m. He was a friend of mine. I was not sure at that time if he had the needed skills (obviously he did), but I knew he had the audacity. I highlighted his username, put the printout in my desk drawer, and forgot about it. Several years later, he approached me and asked if I remembered the incident of the forged letter. He said, rather proudly, that he was the culprit. I opened my drawer and found the printout I had stuck in there a few years back, handing it to him. He was flabbergasted. He said he thought eventually I would be the one to figure it out, but he could not believe that I had said nothing about it in all those years.

One day when I was cleaning up my file directory on the mainframe, which by now had its own disk drive (as opposed to magnetic tape spools), I noticed that I could not open one of my files. I tried editing it, moving it, copying it, even removing it. Nothing worked. This file was somehow inert, and I do not even remember what it was. I suspected it may have been due to a disk-drive error of sorts; perhaps one of the bytes defining the file's header was corrupted on the drive. I was not worried and soon forgot about it. About a year later, a fellow computer-wizard, who may have had hacker aspirations, was boasting that he could access the files of any mainframe user in an hour. I remembered the elusive corrupt file in my home directory. I approached him and told him that I had created a file and left a message in it specifically for him. I gave him the name of the file and told him that I would give him a week to access that file and read the message. I don't remember if there was a bet, but he confidently told me that he would print out the message and bring it to me within the hour. A week later he came and begged me to tell him how I managed to protect that file. He was not as arrogant as he had been a week earlier. I never told him my secret, that it was my wayward corrupt file with no special message to him.

\* \* \*

While I worked hard at both teaching and conducting the compli-cated research for my thesis, life was not all work and no play. (I had learned well from my American students.) On the weekends, Zeynep and I liked to ride our bicycles to explore the city. Fall in Richmond was amazing. The colors of the turning leaves of the old trees along the James River were breathtakingly beautiful, and unlike anything I had ever seen. Going out to eat, which we couldn't afford to do very often, was a real treat. Especially at my favorite New York Delicatessen with their delicious Reuben plate.

I also discovered the chess club at VCU. It was small but well organized. They had tournaments where you played one game a week. Because the tournaments were sanctioned and rated by the United States Chess Federation, each game result led to a rating adjustment. In their system, a rating of 1,500 represents a basic understanding of strategy and tactics, 1,800 is a strong player while 2,000 is an excellent player; 2,200 represented masters and 2,400-plus grandmasters. The first twenty games were provisionally rated so initially my rating fluctuated a lot. It briefly exceeded 2,000 during this period but settled around the 1,800s to 1,900s for the rest of my life—never good enough for a master's level.

Unlike the chess club in Turkey where membership was restricted only to members of the university, the VCU chess club was open and welcomed participants from outside. Still, we organized a tournament open only to VCU affiliates—the faculty, staff, and students of VCU— and I ended up winning it. Later in the year, the club organized an exhibition featuring Edmar Mednis. He was a Latvian grandmaster famous for having beaten Bobby Fisher and then authoring a book entitled *How to Beat Bobby Fisher*. He played against twenty-five of us simultaneously, winning twenty-three of his games very quickly. I was one of two who tied. The event was featured in the local newspaper, including a short interview with me. The article mentioned, erroneously, that I was the VCU champion (based on the tournament result with the VCU affiliates). Some members of the club took issue, saying that VCU champion meant the winner of VCU club tournament that included everyone, not just VCU affiliates. I still feel badly about the inadvertent misrepresentation.

* * *

Zeynep signed up for a master's program in the computer science department and got a part-time job there as a programmer. The job was good news, as we expected to now have enough income to pay the bills with some left to enjoy life. Unfortunately, she had to pay out-of-state tuition, which was twice as much as in-state costs, so most of her income ended up paying her tuition. We had to continue to manage without life's little luxuries.

Meanwhile, I got the news that my father required triple-bypass surgery. I urgently needed to get to Turkey before his operation. My credit card had a $700 limit on it, so I couldn't use it to buy my ticket. I called the bank and explained the situation. They raised the credit card limit to cover the airline ticket, and I flew to Turkey immediately. I was able to see my father a day before the operation, when he seemed in good spirits.

The operation was deemed successful, and he was recovering well. However, now he did not recognize my mother. He kept referring to her by his younger sister's name. The doctors determined he'd had a stroke during or just after the operation. His short-term memory and most of his eyesight was gone. He had to relearn how to read. He could write habitually but would forget the first part of a sentence before he got to the end. He'd been preparing to retire and spend all his time with his stamps. He wouldn't be able to do that anymore. He would ask me what I was doing in America; I would explain. Five minutes later he would ask me the same question again. I was sad to no longer be able to have an adult relationship with my father.

By the time I came back to the US, I'd consumed all of our savings. A new semester was starting, and Zeynep needed to register. By a stroke of luck, the school inadvertently billed Zeynep for in-state tuition since we had been in the city for over a year. So we were able, barely, to cover the cost of registering for the new semester. However, since we were foreign students, we technically weren't considered in-state even after a year of residence. About six weeks later, the university realized their mistake and sent an upwardly revised bill. That six weeks was enough for us to save the necessary money. Phew!

In my second year at VCU, I saw a posting for a fellowship. I quickly applied, seizing upon anything that might reasonably contribute financially to this eternally poor graduate student's coffers. A half dozen other applicants from the department contended in a strict process that included an exam.

I gathered all six of the other students applying and proposed that we study together. Each of us would study one part really well and teach the others the important specifics from that area. This is something we had done a lot in Turkey, but I hadn't seen any such collaborative studying in the US. To my surprise, everyone complied, and we all seemed to be preparing well for the exam. The professors were incredulous. Every ten minutes or so, a faculty member would open the door and look inside, amazed to find us collaborating instead of competing. Several different faculty visited to see this for themselves. We all did well on the exam.

A while after the test, a faculty member visited the lab I was working in and congratulated me for being awarded the "Mary E. Kapp Research Fellowship." I asked him what that meant. He scratched his slightly balding head. "You won't have to teach anymore," he told me. "All your expenses will be covered, and you can now focus on your doctoral research." I was thrilled, of course, but it was bittersweet because I loved teaching. That was the end of my teaching career (except for one organic chemistry class in Alabama during the summer of 1988) until some thirty years later when I would return to teaching at Santa Rosa Junior College post-retirement.

In Turkey, I had written my master's thesis on a typewriter. As older readers with moderate typing skills may remember, it was almost painful to make corrections. So for my doctorate dissertation I used an emerging new software program called LaTeX. It was not yet a "What You See Is What You Get" (WYSIWYG) system, so ubiquitous today, where what you see on the screen is what prints, so I needed to print chapters often to know how they would look. With my words swimming in a sea of computer code on the screen, clean printouts were essential to plan my layout. The big printers lived in a spacious room downstairs in the math department. My constant chapter printing edged out math department students who needed to print. The TAs who maintained the facility started to complain about me using their printers and became somewhat hostile towards me.

Before the time of PCs and personal printers, a certain hierarchy governed access to big mainframe-connected printers, with professors at the top and students at the bottom; graduate students were somewhere in between. So, I can't blame the TAs managing the printer lab for being upset with some graduate student from another department using their precious resources. I, too, was not happy with the situation. By that time, I had a good reputation at the chemistry department, probably due to my research but also with the Math Department probably because of the computational aspects of my work. The Math Department chair must have developed a liking towards me. He gave me the keys to the printer room and told me that I could use the facility anytime I wanted. That solved my problem. I would go downstairs to the printer room after hours and conduct my work in peace and quiet. I finally completed my dissertation towards the end of the fall 1986 semester and was working on revisions. I was tying up loose ends.

One day, a well-respected professor in the department, Dr. Lydia Vallerino, saw me having a coffee in the dining area and asked if she could join me. I welcomed the interruption since I was dealing with dissertation problems, with my mind busy trying to figure out how to prioritize revisions. When you have two supervisors, you have about twice the revisions to make! Dr. Vallerino was a bespeckled older Italian professor liked by all. She had a charming accent. An inorganic chemist, she conducted research that did not overlap much with mine, but she had always been friendly to me.

She said, "Four years earlier, when you were doing your rounds, everybody was interested in recruiting you to their research program as a graduate student. When I interviewed you," she said, "you explained what you wanted to do: experimental and theoretical work that complemented each other." I thought at that time, "This kid is a dreamer. He's flying in the clouds and not realistic in aspiring to do something so complex and difficult. He'll end up having a rough reality check when he actually tries to do it." She continued, "Now, however, I recognize that you ended up doing exactly what you had described to me four years ago and succeeded." This compliment meant a lot to me. Up until then, I had not realized how unusual my project was.

The chemistry department decided to send my dissertation to be considered for a national award: the Nobel Laureate Signature Award. Its purpose is to recognize an outstanding graduate student and his or her preceptor in the field of chemistry as broadly defined. The American Chemical Society selects one doctorate project for this award every year; the winning faculty supervisor and the graduate student are recognized as the publishers of the top dissertation in the US that year. I didn't stand a chance, of course, since the competition would be from top universities with top funding and top professors. It turned out that such a nomination had never been made in the history of the graduate program at VCU. So they had to come up with a process. One aspect of the process, they decided, was to have the dissertation reviewed by an external professor with expertise in the field. I did not follow the progress of the application much, but I saw the incredibly supportive letter from the external professor. He wrote that he had worked in several Ivy League universities, and this dissertation would be considered successful at any of them. This was important validation for me. My dissertation did not win the prize, but I was thrilled to have been nominated, a nice closure to my graduate work. All my academic accomplishments continued to surprise me and my low self-esteem. Perhaps I could now develop more confidence in my future abilities. Perhaps I should take more chances and move out of my comfort zone. I mentally decided to work in on this.

Meanwhile, Zeynep became pregnant. We had avoided pregnancy, earlier, during my doctorate and Zeynep's master's. We didn't think raising a baby during the rush of studies and with relatively uncertain finances was a good idea. But now that the doctorate was over, I would be getting a postdoctoral salary and benefits so we could afford to start a family. Zeynep didn't have time to finish her master's degree, but the department offered to graduate her with a certificate, enough for her to work as a programmer analyst in the future.

I started looking for postdoctoral opportunities. While my master's project was fully experimental, my PhD was half experimental and half theoretical. I wanted my postdoctoral project to be entirely theoretical. I would smoothly transition from experimental bench work to theoretical computational work. Instead of working in a wet chemistry lab pouring solutions from flasks to reaction vessels, I would work in a computer lab.

It didn't take me long to find an opportunity. The University of Alabama at Birmingham had a postdoctoral fellowship position involving quantum mechanical calculations in search for new materials to be used as rocket propellants. It sounded fascinating.

# CHAPTER 5

# Postdoctoral Fellowship
# at UAB

## *Birmingham, Alabama, 1987-1989*

Postdoctoral work is like the honeymoon of an academic career.

- During graduate school you do research—the fun part—but you also must consider grades, classes, and your dissertation.
- During your professorship you get to do research—the fun part —but you also worry about classes, grant proposals, committee meetings, and tenure requirements.
- During your postdoc, however, you do research, and that is it. You can always do more, but you are required to do the fun part first.

So, I was looking forward to starting my career honeymoon at University of Alabama at Birmingham (UAB).

\* \* \*

On the first of January 1987, I arrived in Birmingham, Alabama to start my postdoctoral fellowship with a shiny new PhD in physical organic chemistry. To help with our finances, Zeynep decided to stay one more month in Richmond to continue with her job in the computer science department. Since she was no longer paying tuition, her entire last paycheck would go into our savings. I would return to Richmond a month later and we would lease a U-Haul trailer and drive back to Birmingham together.

I leased one of the apartments reserved for staff and faculty, a five-minute walk from work. At work, the space designated for the computational chemistry lab was not ready, so I settled into a small corner of a large room that was occupied by the glass blower (who provided custom glassware for the research projects that needed them) and his equipment; the opposite corner was also used temporarily as an overflow meeting room. I created the foundation for a small cubicle surrounding my corner with narrow tables. A MicroVAX-II computer[3] on which I would begin my work dominated the center of the cubicle. The computational lab relied on VAX computers running the VAX/VMS operating system, much as the IBM mainframes ran the UNIX operating system at VCU. First order of business: I would have to learn the new (to me) VAX/VMS operating system by reading the twentysix volumes of the manual. These thick tomes, stacked on my narrow tables, also served well as walls for my makeshift cubicle.

My postdoctoral project was part of a twenty-year United States Air Force (USAF) research initiative, funded in five-year chunks. Someone must have noticed that, despite many advances in space technology, the rocket propellants used at that time were decades old with no recent fuel innovations. So, the initiative sought to discover new fuel technologies for rockets. The project dedicated the first five years, which we were in the midst of, to theory—the complex, mathematically driven science that was my playground. Testing actual compounds would come later. We were among a dozen or so institutions (including government agencies, academic universities, and industrial institutions) pursuing this theoretical part of the initiative.

My boss, Dr. Koop Lammertsma, proposed funding from this initiative to theoretically identify new high energy/high density materials. His successful proposal made my postdoctoral fellowship possible.

Dr. Lammertsma had white-streaked curly brown hair, a full beard, and a mustache. Well recognized in the quantum chemistry world, he collaborated with some of the most respected figures in both theoretical and experimental chemistry. He had an experimental lab where students synthesized actual (as opposed to theoretical) compounds. Now he was founding the computational lab, and I would be its first scientist.

I lacked all the details for the big picture, but my job was clear. We would develop "potential energy hypersurfaces" of small "tetraatomic" molecular clusters. Tetraatomic means a molecule with only four atoms. Though they're termed clusters because in reality innumerable identically structured four-atom molecules exist together; my work examined the theoretical behavior of individual tetratomic molecules. Such a molecule can attain different conformations (subatomic configurations—determined by how the atom's electrons are behaving) and can move from one conformation to another by overcoming an energy barrier. Each configuration it might attain also represents a specific energy level for the molecule.

Imagine a ball-rolling game you might see at a county fair; something like in the picture next page (which is actually a screen shot of a computer game). When you roll the ball, you are supplying it with kinetic energy. If this energy is enough to push it over the ridge, it may settle into the lowest point in the next well.

Now imagine that the ball is your molecule, and the curved surface represents the potential energy hypersurface. The bottom of each well represents the most stable configurations and, thus, the lowest energy conformations for the molecule. In the game, the ridges and their low saddle points that the ball needs to traverse to get to the next dip are energy barriers that the ball must overcome. Similarly, ridges and saddles on a potential energy hypersurface define the amount of energy that must be applied for the molecule to go over the barrier to the next valley—to get from one stable, low-energy configuration to another. In the figure, the small blue circle represents just enough energy for the ball (i.e., molecule) to go over the ridge to settle in the first well. The larger blue circle represents the amount of energy needed for it go over the larger barrier.

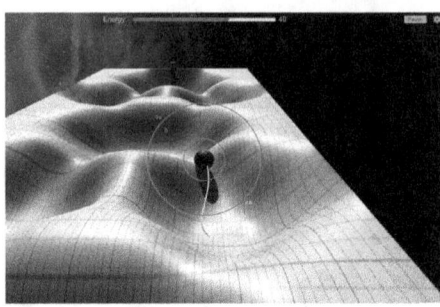

**Depiction of a molecule moving around a potential energy hypersurface.**
*http://atomicconceptssoftware.appspot.com/ SmoothRollerWebSite/smooth_roller.html Copyright © 2019 Atomic Concepts Software*

We would generate this potential energy hypersurface for each of our tetraatomic molecules using quantum mechanical (QM) calculations to determine the lowest point energies at the bottom of a well (i.e., minimum energy conformation of a molecule) and the energy needed to go over to the next well (i.e., the magnitude of the blue spheres in the figure). We would perform QM calculations for developing the hypersurfaces starting with low levels of theory to get the initial three-dimensional (3D) structures of the minimum energy conformations of various arrangement of the atoms in the clusters. These minimum energy structures represent stable conformations of the molecule.

Using those minimum energy structures, we would repeat the calculations, gradually increasing the levels of theory to improve our results, getting our theoretical calculations to ever more closely predict reality. Levels of theory vary the complexity of the basis sets we used in calculations. The more complex, the higher the levels of theory, and the exponentially higher the central processing unit (CPU) and memory requirements.[4] Hence, higher levels of theory will produce better quality and more reliable results but cost significantly more in resources. My boss already had some half a dozen small tetraatomic clusters in mind to start my work, so my job was clearly defined.

Soon, I understood the VAX/VMS operating system well enough, and with OPER privilege (a high-level system privilege that allows the operator to create and control all queues), I could line up QM calculations and prioritize them so that the CPU would never stay idle, thereby achieving maximum efficiency. I would line up several jobs at each computer and, as they were completed, I would add more jobs, making sure that each computer always had several jobs waiting in line.

As soon as one job was finished, the next one in the queue would start automatically with no lapse in CPU usage.

Over time, our computational lab facilities were completed, including a huge cooling system that kept us so cool during summer that we had to keep winter clothing handy. I had an office with a desk holding a VAX workstation, and some added table space to line up all the printouts from completed jobs. This was a significant improvement over the makeshift cubicle carved into a corner of the glass blower's lab. In fact, this was the first time I had an office of my own. It was right next to my boss's office, and two more smaller offices awaited future tenants.

We started with a network of five VAX workstations running day and night thanks to my relentless scheduling. When a VAX maintenance person came to the lab for the computers' scheduled six-month maintenance, he was dumbfounded when he saw that the CPU usage on all five computers was one hundred percent for the entire six months. He said he had never seen such a thing in his career as a VAX maintenance operator.

Once the facility was completed, the office spaces started filling up. An Indian graduate student, Sudhakar, and a Polish postdoctoral fellow, Jerzy, joined the group. They were both exceptionally good scientists. Sudhakar worked part time on the USAF initiative, and we ended up coauthoring several papers together. Jerzy was working in a different area, so I did not have much scientific interaction with him. Then a Dutch graduate student, Mark, joined the group. He was enthusiastic about computers, so my boss decided to employ him as the information technology (IT) manager for our lab to give him some financial support. Our facility had grown with some added minicomputers and early PCs, and he felt it could use a devoted person to support it. Mark learned the job quickly, and the systems were running smoothly and efficiently. It seemed like our boss made the right decision to hire an IT manager.

One morning when I came into the office, I noticed that one of my big jobs that had been running for over a week had stopped, and I was not able to revive it. This had never happened before. I panicked, and at once ran to my boss's office so that we could investigate what happened, and to see if we might salvage the job. My boss had full system privileges so he could explore all the details of why the job had stopped and when. It turned out that the IT manager had been watching the system late the previous night. One of my jobs was hogging resources (memory and CPU), pushing the limits of our capacity. Not realizing that this had been our modus operandi since the lab's beginning, he decided to terminate my job. But he didn't stop there; he also decided to take away my OPER privileges so that I would not be able to load the system as much anymore.

My boss was furious. He said, "Everything in this lab is being funded by the work that you are doing. The work must continue with maximum efficiency and with the highest priority as it has been so far." He at once reinstated my OPER privileges and told me to continue the research the way I was doing it. He was done; the decision was made with his pragmatism on full display. I do not know what Mark's conversation with the boss was about, because I never saw Mark again. I soon found out that he left our group and joined one in the biology department to continue with his doctorate.

What happened with Mark was not uncommon, especially in larger institutions. In general, IT groups would typically be established as a service organization, enabling its clientele to perform the important work of the institution. After a while, sometimes IT managers get used to their power and authority and transform into gatekeepers instead of service providers. Their desire to keep the network running smoothly can lead them to take an overly cautious approach and enforce needless rules at the expense of the institution's essential existential work.

* * *

Zeynep was getting bigger. We started putting together the bag with all the items we'd need to bring with us to the hospital for childbirth. We would take walks around the campus. The UAB hospital was within walking distance of our place, and they had just constructed a new "maternity pavilion." We stopped by the hospital to tour the new pavilion, and her doctor wanted to check Zeynep's progress while we were there. Good thing, because her water was about to break, and they decided to check her in. I rushed home to pick up the ready bag and went back to the hospital.

She was in her room, which appeared no different from a regular living room, with a couch, a couple of chairs, a television set, and nice paintings hanging on the walls. However, one drawer of the nightstand held some of the instruments that would be used to monitor stats like heartbeat and oxygen saturation. The wall paintings hid connections for medical necessities like oxygen. An area in the corner partitioned off all sorts of other equipment on wheels. The living room could be converted into an operating room within minutes if needed. The set up was at once luxurious and medically advanced. Zeynep's treatment was fully covered by our UAB healthcare benefit. Our son, Kurt, made his entrance in this environment almost like royalty. I was there the whole time holding Zeynep's hand. Witnessing childbirth was an amazing experience. After his umbilical cord was cut, Kurt was whisked away for his circumcision. Even though we were secular, we decided to abide by this Moslem/Jewish tradition. Zeynep, looked exhausted but ecstatic. I was slowly coming to realize that our lives had irreversibly changed, as this small, helpless individual would rely on us for his survival.

* * *

At one point, Dr. Lammertsma offered me a side project. His former postdoctoral supervisor, Dr. George Olah, a top experimental scientist, needed theoretical validation of a project his team was working on. He said I could run high-level quantum mechanical calculations to supplement their experimental work, and we would publish a quick paper on this project. This sounded fine. In academia, the number and quality of one's publications contribute to a scientist's advancement, particularly to their ability to attain tenure and attract funding. I had not yet decided on an academic or corporate career, but either way it would help to have additional publications coauthored with top scientists in my *curriculum vitae* (CV, a scientist's version of a resume that can run several pages long and list dozens, even hundreds, of the scientist's published works).

It took me a couple of weeks to run the calculations and send the results and my analysis to the two professors. Shortly thereafter, the *Journal of the American Chemical Society* (*JACS*) published it.[5] The earlier few papers I had published at *JACS,* one of the hardest journals in which to get published, had faced serious scrutiny. My coauthors and I went back and forth with the reviewers for months before they accepted our paper. This time, however, to my surprise, our paper was accepted as is. I never thought this was possible with *JACS*. George Olah must have been a very influential scientist to get his papers accepted so quickly. And indeed, he was. Several years later he received a Nobel Prize in Chemistry.

About a decade or so later I attended the National Awards Ceremony when I was working for Accelrys, which sponsored a major industry award. Unbeknownst to me, George Olah was receiving another award, the Priestly Medal, one of the most prestigious awards in chemistry (after the Nobel Prize). After he received the award, I approached to congratulate him. Though we were coauthors of a paper, this was the first time I had met him in person. He took a careful look at my name badge, but I saw no recognition in his eyes. I think I may have bragging rights to having coauthored a paper with a Nobel Laureate—who never knew I existed.

About a year after the project with Dr. Olah completed, my boss approached me again asking if I could contribute to another collaboration, this time with Dr. John Pople. I declined because I did not think I had enough time left for side projects anymore. I was trying to complete my calculations since I was approaching the end of my postdoctoral funding. I would come to regret that decision as Dr. Pople received his Nobel Prize a few years after Dr. Olah did. It would have been nice for me to have a paper with Dr. Pople as well. Maybe he would have even known who I was.

\* \* \*

During May 1987, Dr. Lammertsma and I attended the first High Energy Density Matter (HEDM) Conference in Virginia, organized by the Air Force Astronautics Laboratory. It was good to see all the other people working on this project and hear firsthand their challenges and advances. My boss delivered a paper he and I had published on the second day of the conference. This was the first major scientific conference I had ever attended (excepting some small local events), and I learned a lot. Even though conference participation was restricted to the contractors of the USAF initiative, the level of scientific innovation pushing the frontiers forward was intriguing. I was thrilled to be a part of such an initiative.

One of the highlights of this trip, for me, was our visit to the National Gallery of Art in Washington, DC. My boss and I thoroughly enjoyed the visit and all the art from Europe's Renaissance. Many works by Dutch artists stoked Dr. Lammertsma's pride in his nationality. At one point, he asked how come he hadn't seen any Turkish art? I was struggling to come up with an answer; perhaps that the Ottoman art scene had peaked at an earlier time. But once we turned the corner, I didn't have to answer at all. The special exhibit entitled "The Age of Sultan Süleyman the Magnificent," answered for me. We paid the additional fee to enter. The exhibit didn't have many paintings and sculptures, but it displayed ancient manuscripts, kaftans, embroideries, rugs, ceramics, and imperial items of gold and silver embellished with gems from the Ottoman period, and it evoked my own pride of heritage.

\* \* \*

The Alabama Supercomputer Center was being set up at Huntsville in 1988 while I was doing my postdoctoral work. It was about three miles from the Huntsville campus of the University of Alabama and about seven miles from the Marshall Space Center, the US government's civilian rocketry and spacecraft propulsion research center. The historic Redstone Rocket Test Site also neighbored the Marshall Space Center. Huntsville is where Dr. Wernher Von Braun developed the Saturn V rocket used in the moon shots. The center would house a then-ultramodern Cray supercomputer, and Boeing would be managing the Center.

Experienced with the process, Boeing people knew that once the supercomputer was online, in the beginning it would sit practically idle.

Projects take time to build up, especially on a supercomputer where the results come in so fast, scientists end up spending most of their time analyzing results before submitting the next job. To speed the ramp-up process, about a month before the new system came online, Boeing administrators gave us an account on their existing supercomputer in Seattle (the one, I suspect, they used some years later to design the parts for the Boeing 777 airplane, the first computer-aided designed airplane). This way, we could start working on our projects in Seattle, and once the Huntsville supercomputer was up and running, transfer our ramped-up jobs to the Cray. Apparently, they had done this before and learned that the fastest way to get a supercomputer busy is to set loose a couple of theoretical chemists running QM calculations on it. We toyed with the challenge of increasing the level of theory or increasing the size of the molecules to bring the supercomputer to its knees with the massively complex calculations required (but we exhibited restraint).

Access to a supercomputer was great. A job that would take a week running on our VAX network of computers would only take an hour on a Cray. And because the system was not used to full capacity, the administrators were generous with the allocation of computer time to eligible scientists in Alabama. It would only take a half-page proposal to secure several hours of assigned Cray time. Eventually, within about a year, the Cray got to full capacity as all the universities in Alabama started using it. The load was not being effectively managed, however. Jobs were not prioritized based on how long they would take. The jobs we sent would end up waiting in queue for about a week—then be completed within an hour. So, it became barely worth running our jobs on the Cray. We could run them on our VAX machines for a week and get the same results in just about the same time. So, we started saving our Cray use for exceptionally large jobs.

\* \* \*

I continued with my physical and cerebral hobbies during my post-doc. UAB had a small chess club where I participated in tournaments, but chess was no longer a priority activity for me. Volleyball, however, still enamored me, and I regularly played pickup games. Once

I participated in a two-on-two tournament. This is much like beach volleyball in the Olympic games but played on a full-sized volleyball court. So a large space had to be covered by only two people leading to excessive (in my mind) running around. And unlike in beach volleyball, when you dove, you could easily get hurt. This activity did provide the cardiovascular exercise I needed.

We celebrated Kurt's first birthday in June 1988. Kurt had long black eyelashes. Whenever we went out for a walk with him in his stroller, people would stop us to comment on those eyelashes.

He was a cautious baby. We tried to encourage him to walk, but he wouldn't leave the safety of holding someone's hand or clutching the side of a couch. During his birthday party, other children about his age were walking around. So Kurt just stood up and started to walk on his own. That was it. All he had needed was to see other kids his age walking.

* * *

In the summer of 1988, my boss was in Germany working with an associate, Dr. Paul Schleyer at the University of Erlangen. Dr. Schleyer was one of the heavy-weights in theoretical chemistry, much like Dr. Olah is one of the heavy-weights in experimental chemistry. They each had over 800 publications at that time. Dr. Schleyer had visited our lab a few months prior. From the discussions that culminated from this meeting, Dr. Lammertsma and I ended up collaborating on two projects that resulted in two papers we coauthored.[6,7]

As the senior member of the group, I was delegated the responsibility of managing the computational chemistry lab in Dr. Lammertsma's absence. My boss would have weekly conference calls with me to go over the projects and deal with any issues that had arisen during the week. So I was going to be, almost, my own boss for a couple of months that summer.

In the interim, the chemistry department chair asked if I would be willing to teach an organic chemistry class during the summer semester, an offer I enthusiastically accepted. The additional stipend was welcome, as any extra money helped with the expenses of raising one-year-old Kurt. But more importantly, I would be teaching: an activity I loved to do. Meanwhile, because I still had access to computer time on the Cray, I decided to come up with a short side project that I could complete during the summer to explore developing projects on my own in case I decided to stay in academia. I searched the literature carefully to find cases where experimental results and theoretical calculations conflicted with each other. With access to a Cray, I could take the QM calculations to much higher levels of theory than other people were able to and perhaps resolve the conflict and publish the results more quickly than they could.

I found one such case. Some of Dr. William Lipscomb's work on boron chemistry was one of the cases where the experimental results and theoretical predictions disagreed. (Dr. Lipscomb was the 1976 Chemistry Nobel Laureate.) I started by repeating the calculations that were already published. Once I verified them, I had a baseline set up from which I could take the calculations to much higher levels to see if the predictions would reverse. I was discussing this with my boss during one of our weekly conference calls, and he said that Dr. Schleyer asked "what is Osman trying to do that Lipscomb had not already done?"

I checked all the literature and reviewed several of Dr. Lipscomb's relevant papers, and he had not done the calculations at the levels I was proposing. I was perplexed until.... In the next issue of *JACS*, Dr. Lipscomb indeed published a paper in which he performed the calculations close to the levels I was planning. The predictions *were* reversed and now the theory and experiment agreed with each other. I was scooped—but I was happy that at least I was scooped by a Nobel Laureate refining his own work. Meanwhile, I was wondering, how had Schleyer known about Lipscomb's paper before it was published? Was he a reviewer for that paper, or did he have early access to the journal? At any rate, the summer project did not pan out, but at least I confirmed I could develop a credible research program on my own.

\* \* \*

In September 1988, I took part in my first American Chemical Society (ACS) National meeting. With an average attendance of 20,000 to

30,000 people, ACS National meetings constitute the largest gathering of chemists around the world. The twice-a-year meetings would alternate between the East or West side of the US. This meeting was in Los Angeles. We stayed in the Westin Bonaventure Hotel (my first stay in a posh hotel). I was overly ambitious and showed off by presenting papers in four different divisions.[8]

I was also approaching the end of my postdoctoral fellowship, so wanted to investigate some of the software companies in the chemistry field as potential employers. I figured having worked in the US would help me with my job applications in Turkey later. But I also wanted to keep available the option to emigrate to the US permanently. At ACS, they had a job fair inside the exposition area where you could make appointments with various employers. I didn't see too many opportunities of interest to me, but one position seemed relevant. Molecular Design Limited (MDL) was looking for an application scientist to market their new 3D information management software. I made an appointment and met with the Human Resources (HR) director. The position was mildly interesting, but I was thinking of passing since it didn't involve QM calculations. But I gathered the forms, mainly so that I wouldn't return from the meeting empty-handed.

The job market was tight and required some effort and planning to find suitable jobs prospects and apply. The Air Force Astronautics Laboratory wanted me to continue work on rocket propellants at the Edwards Air Force Base in California. This famous site is where test pilots put many new Air Force and NASA planes through their paces. They sent me several forms for the employment application process. At about the same time, Boeing also showed interest in hiring me. They wanted to recruit me for a position at the Huntsville Supercomputer Center.

I had an offer for a second postdoctoral appointment from Dr. Corwin Hansch at Pomona College. He had been alerted to my track record of prolific QM calculations and needed someone to generate new descriptors for quantitative structure-activity relationship (QSAR) models. Structure activity relationship (SAR) analysis had been in use for a long time in drug design, specifically during the lead optimization process (when researchers seek the best molecular candidates to test as potential drugs). Making small, incremental changes in the molecular structure, and testing how each small change affects the molecule's activity, let scientists develop a sense for the type of structural features responsible for a specific biological effect. QSAR is the quantitative version of this concept, providing a mathematical model to predict the activity of compounds. Not knowing people outside of my immediate field, I didn't realize that Dr. Hansch was a big shot. Sensing my hesitancy, he mailed me a packet with some of his papers and the list of citations he received in the previous year. It was amazing. Just one of his papers had more than several thousand citations in the previous year alone.[9] I didn't know it at that time, but he was considered the father of QSAR.

Meanwhile, the only job application I had made at the ACS job fair resulted in an interview invitation from MDL for an applications scientist position. The night before my trip to San Francisco for the interview, I received a phone call from my Boeing liaison offering me ten percent more than any MDL offer.

I was feeling particularly good about myself. The interview went okay. At the end of the day, I mentioned some of the possible job considerations I had to the HR person who took note of them and excused himself to consult someone. When he returned a few minutes later, he told me that they would be in touch; meanwhile I should enjoy my weekend in San Francisco, all expenses paid. This was my first trip to the San Francisco Bay Area, and I had fallen in love with the city at once. A few months later, I received a job offer from MDL. They wanted me to start in June as a "senior" applications scientist. "Senior?" I ended up getting promoted even before I started the job. I guess they wanted to match the approximate salary range I was entertaining with competing offers.

Back in Alabama I was conflicted. What to do? Which one to pick? Each of the opportunities would put me on a different career path, and my life would be vastly different with each job. If I took the Air Force offer, I would start a career working at government labs. If I took the Boeing offer, I would become a glorified IT manager, and spend all my time with computers. If I took the second postdoc position with Dr. Hansch, I would likely end up with an academic position. If I took the job at MDL, I would have to switch fields from material science to life sciences, an area of which I was ignorant.

I was at a critical juncture, facing probably the most consequential decision of my life up to that point. I was suffering from "analysis paralysis." But I needed to decide soon.

While struggling with these choices, I had a dream. A small girl of about five with long, wavy, dark hair, apparently my future grand-daughter, was asking me what I had done with my life. I was struggling with an answer, trying to explain that I was helping people develop better explosives. How could I put a positive spin on that? With this struggle, I woke up clearly remembering the dream, which encouraged me to look at the big picture of each of my choices. By the time I was out of my shower, I had made one decision. It would either be MDL, or a second postdoc with Dr. Hansch.

Meanwhile, we found out that Zeynep was pregnant with our second child. It was time to get a real job with real money and bene-fits, so that eliminated the second postdoc option. I was going to San Francisco, switching to life sciences, and starting over (again). Inciden-tally, two days later, the Boeing offer was retracted because I was not an American citizen.

# CHAPTER 6

# At MDL

*San Leandro, California, 1989-1996*

Starting my first "real" job in the US, I was excited. Molecular Design Limited (MDL) was the leading company supplying chemical information management systems to the chemical and pharmaceutical industries. MDL's flagship product was *MACCS-II* (MACCS stands for Molecular ACCess System). They were expanding their software solutions to encompass three-dimensional (3D) structures with *MACCS-3D*. I was to support this expansion.

Being able to represent the specific shapes that a molecule may hold in 3D space and record those various possible shapes in a searchable database is a valuable pharmaceutical research tool. By establishing the physical arrangements in space of the features of molecules with known biological activity, scientists can create a 3D template—called a "pharmacophore model." They can use that model to search a database of 3D structures for other molecules with similarly shaped portions that may mimic the model and induce a similar biological response.

Consider a lock and a key, where the lock is the biological receptor in the body (often found on the surface of specific cells of interest) and the key is the molecule scientists want to mimic because of its known biological activity when it interacts with the receptor—with the lock. But perhaps that key, the known molecule, also unlocks another receptor, causing an undesired effect, a toxic side effect. Or perhaps it is bulky and thus too difficult to get into the body. So, scientists may want to find a molecule that has a similar enough shape to also unlock the desired receptor/lock, but that is different enough to not interact with receptors that cause side effects; or that is smaller overall and easier to administer.

Appendix I provides a good example. To establish the 3D arrangement of a desired molecule's features, scientists used the 3D structure of a ligand (key) that is bound to the receptor (lock) and that induces the desired biological effect. By fixing these features in 3D space, and removing the extraneous portions of the molecule, scientists obtain a pharmacophore model with which to search databases to retrieve compounds that match the 3D arrangement of the features of the pharmacophore. Some of these retrieved novel compounds may make attractive new drug candidates.

While the mechanical lock-and-key metaphor may help to understand how this works, especially when considering traditional two-dimensional chemical structures, it is actually a bit too simplistic when looking at molecules in 3D space, because molecular shapes as we perceive them can be deceiving. The ligand-receptor interaction is really more akin to an electronic key.

Imagine looking at and enjoying a landscape in the evening. Now put on infrared goggles and see what appears to be a different landscape. It is the same landscape, but now you perceive it differently. The landscape is now color coded with respect to the heat temperature of the objects. It looks different to us because our naked eyes see only a small sliver of the broad electromagnetic frequency range. The approximately 2% of electromagnetic radiation that we see is called visible light (violet on the high energy side and red on the low energy side, with the remaining rainbow of colors ranging in between). Further out on the higher energy spectrum, a bit beyond our visible violet color, you enter the ultraviolet (UV) region. Here, we humans can no longer see the light, but we can feel the evidence of it, like a sunburn after staying under the sun for too long. If we move toward the lower energy spectrum, slightly beyond our visible red, we enter the infrared (IR) region; again, we cannot see it, but here we can feel the evidence of it as heat. Now, consider that the vision of some animals is across a broader spectrum than of human vision. For example, vipers can see IR light. If a viper stalks prey, say a rat, hiding behind a bush, it can see right through the bush and locate the not-so-well-hidden rat based on its heat signature.

Now, let's apply this concept to pharmacophores. We humans have developed a chemistry convention to recognize and differentiate chemical compounds. For example, we represent carbon with the letter C, oxygen with the letter O, and hydrogen with the letter H. We can then represent a water molecule as $H_2O$—a molecule with two hydrogen atoms attached to an oxygen atom.

Similarly, we have drug molecules with lots of carbons, oxygens, and hydrogens. What does the receptor (the lock) see in such a molecule? It does not see carbons, oxygens, or hydrogens, as these represent a convention we created to make things easy for ourselves. Rather, it sees (or feels) the abstract features of a molecule in 3D space: here is an electron-rich region that can supply electrons, and there is an electron-poor region that can accept electrons, etc. To represent our drug molecules closer to the way the receptor enzyme sees them, we construct a pharmacophore model of the drug molecule. For example, we look at two molecules that look completely different with our standard conventions, but if we put on our pharmacophore goggles, suddenly they seem similar, as the 3D arrangement of their electron population is similar despite how their atoms are arranged in our molecular models.

With our pharmacophore model based on an active compound (or a series of them), we can search the chemical databases to retrieve compounds that match the model without necessarily having similar structural features. By doing so, we may be able to identify a novel compound that the receptor perceives to be similar enough to the active compounds (just as the viper perceives the rat right through the bush). The resulting molecules represent potential new drugs that may be structurally different than those already known. Because they are structurally different than the active molecule we started with, they may sidestep issues of our initial active compounds, such as toxic side effects, or problems with delivering the molecule into the body. One of the new active compounds may not be toxic, because it is structurally different than the known active compounds. Or it may be smaller than the known active compound. But in pharmacophore space, the way the receptor enzyme sees them, they may be quite similar. The electronic key fits the electronic lock, even if, to us, it looks quite different than the original key, say like a card or a fob, instead of like a classic key.

The most recent definition recommended by the International Union of Pure and Applied Chemistry (IUPAC) states:[10] "A pharmacophore is the ensemble of steric and electronic features that is necessary to ensure the optimal supramolecular interactions with a specific biological target structure and to trigger (or to block) its biological response."

The emerging 3D information management technology would provide scientists the ability to develop pharmacophore models; as such, it could bring about a paradigm shift in drug discovery.[11] For those interested in learning more about how this technology is used in drug discovery, I recommend a short article I authored, published in *Investigational Drugs*, specifically designed to explain the concept for non-specialist scientists.[12]

* * *

As I engaged with my job, I noted vast differences from the academic work environment. First, everything was fast. Most activities had deadlines. People ran meetings more efficiently.

Because I was championing a new technology, I traveled for business quite a bit, a new experience for me. With my Turkish passport, traveling overseas was cumbersome. I needed visas for most of the destination countries. Typically, a trip to Europe would involve visiting clients in several different countries. I needed to get visas for each country in reverse order of visiting, since each country wanted to see my visa for my next destination before allowing me entry. This was before the European Union, so just one visa did not cut it.

Once I was traveling to Basel, Switzerland, where MDL's European headquarters was located. My flight connected through Paris. When I attempted to transfer to my flight to Basel, I was told I needed a visa to complete my trip. Basel airport has Swiss, French, and German sections as the city spreads around the borders with each country. It turned out that my connection from Paris to Basel was on a French domestic flight (as opposed to an international flight due to an error made by my travel agent), so I needed a French visa since I would technically be traveling within France. They were friendly and issued me a temporary transit visa so that I could finish the first leg of my trip. They urged me, however, to go to the French consulate in Basel and get a regular visa before my trip back to the US connecting through Paris. Obediently, I went to the French consulate in Basel to get my visa. The officer there said that I did not need a visa since I was not going into France, but just transiting through the airport. I insisted they issue me a visa as the French officers in Paris had warned I needed one. The consular official wouldn't budge. Then I asked her to "Please write down the reasons you aren't going to issue me a visa on an official paper with consulate letterhead so that I can produce it if I have a problem at the airport." She did. I don't speak French, so I didn't know the contents, but I pocketed the letter and went about my business. On the day of my departure, as expected, I was asked to show my visa. I explained how the consulate had insisted I didn't need a visa. The agent was saying "yeah, yeah, I have heard this before," very condescendingly, assuming that I was making this up. So, I handed him the letter. As he started reading it, his face went from pink, to red, to crimson by the time he finished. He apologized and asked to have my passport, went to the French side, then came back five minutes later with a transit visa on my passport.

Sometimes this visa situation put me in an awkward position with my colleagues. Once, when I was in Basel for a few days towards the end of the year, the international colleagues with whom I had been working said that they had scheduled a surprise New Year's party and dinner for the employees of the Basel office, and I was going to be the guest of honor. When the day came, I found out that the surprise party was to be held at a classy restaurant on the French side of Basel. I explained to them that I would not be able to join them since I did not have a visa for France, but that they should have fun and celebrate a successful completion of the year without me. Because a venue switch to the Swiss side at that celebratory time of year was not feasible, they celebrated without me, and I ate alone in my hotel room.

Most Americans don't appreciate the hassle we have to go through for these seemingly routine trips. Each trip must be rigorously planned, the visas acquired, with no room for flexibility if a last-minute change in the itinerary, for instance, to visit a client in Frankfurt on my way to London, was required.

Apart from the hassle to get all the visas sorted out, I enjoyed traveling around the world and experiencing different cultures, different lifestyles, different business processes. I was also making more money, and Zeynep, Kurt and I could now enjoy living in a better neighborhood, driving better cars, dining out, going on excursions, and traveling for holidays.

The amazing corporate culture at MDL valued its employees. Every Friday afternoon, the whole company would go to the San Leandro Marina for a company sponsored picnic. MDL had exceeded its growth goals for twenty-four consecutive quarters before it went public as MDL Information Systems in 1993. So, working for a successful company, I experienced an entirely different mood and work environment, one I have not seen in many other companies.

My time there was an intense learning experience, not only for new science, but also for how to function at a profit-based company under exceptional leadership. MDL also sponsored me for a green card, which took about five years to get. With it, travel became easier at airports, though I still needed visas for the countries I was to visit. I truly enjoyed my tenure at MDL. I had a satisfactory seven years of employment that ended well, but I still remember occasional stressful situations.

After we released *MACCS-3D* towards the end of 1989, our team worked to develop a marketing disk that would be freely distributed to prospects to demonstrate the benefits of the new software system.

This was before the internet, social media, and cell phones. We were to distribute the material on a 3½-inch floppy disk. I developed the PC version of the disk, and two other people developed the Macintosh version. At a certain place in the demo, I used a storyboard software program to rotate a molecule 360 degrees. It provided the wow moment of the scenario the disk was describing. Software limitations prevented the team working on the Mac version from doing this rotation. This should have been okay as the two versions did not have to be identical if the message remained the same. However, the Mac team lobbied for me to remove the rotation. To my surprise, my boss relented to the pressure and decided that I should remove the spiffy rotating molecule. He reasoned that "the 3D rotation would give the impression that the users could do 3D manipulations with the software, and that would mislead the prospects." I was shocked. The name of the software had 3D in it and that was okay, yet having an attractive 3D rotation in the disk could mislead our prospective clients?

My boss's decision to downgrade one version of the demo disk was, in my view, a mistake. He was my first supervisor in the industrial setting, and I looked up to him. After this incident, however, I lost some of my respect for him. An account representative who took part in the project later came to me and asked for a copy of the disk with 3D rotation. He said he would use it when he was personally showing it to the prospects.

* * *

One thing that helped avoid boredom during my business trips was chess. If I was staying someplace over the weekend, I would find a local chess tournament in which to participate. During one of these trips, security officers stopped me at the airport security checkpoint and searched my bags. They were concerned about the way my chess clock looked when scanned. Perhaps, they thought it was a part for a time bomb. Trying to incorporate chess into my busy life became increasingly cumbersome. After a while, it was taking too much time, and I decided to stop playing the game. But I needed to do something to fill the cerebral void. So, I decided to give backgammon a try.

I learned how to play backgammon when I was a kid in Turkey where it's popular, so I knew how the pieces, which are checkers, moved. When I started to play in the US years later, I was surprised to see that the game was being played with a doubling cube, which made it an entirely different game.

Backgammon is a two-player game where each player has fifteen checkers that move between twenty-four spaces according to the roll of two dice. The objective of the game is to be first to bear off, i.e., move all fifteen pieces off the board.

The doubling cube offers the opponent a choice to accept the cube, after which the game will be double-scored, or to reject the cube and instantly lose the point. If the opponent accepts the cube, that person will own the cube with a worth of two points to whoever wins (instead of the usual one point for a game), and at an opportune time has the option of turning it to a worth of four points. Now if the original player accepts the cube, the game will be worth four points to whoever wins. Rejecting it is only desirable if you anticipate losing and want to minimize the opponents' score.

With the doubling cube, in addition to good checker play, one must develop a sense for figuring out the equity of both players' boards during the game to assess whether it is time to turn the doubling cube. During every game there is a window of equity distribution when it is *correct* to double, and the opponent is *correct* to accept the cube. Once past this window, the opponent will likely decline the cube, and you will settle for a one-point win, missing the opportunity to win two points. If the cube is turned too early, however, the opponent will accept the cube and have the advantage of cube ownership and, following a good roll, can turn the cube from two to four. In short, one needs to have a good understanding of cube play to be competitive in backgammon.

So, I had a bit of learning to go through to be competitive. I studied, learned, experimented with ideas, and developed a skill set that would put me at an above average level. This meant I would occasionally win local tournaments, but mostly finish around the middle of the pack. I could never master the equity calculation of each player's board at a given point, making my timing for turning the cube usually a bit off. I also couldn't count the pips fast enough (the number of steps each of the checkers is away from bearing off) to figure out who was ahead in the race. Later, I invented a technique to approximate the pip count that would give me just enough information about the race to help make informed decisions during the game. Without good cube play, I could never be a master level player in backgammon. But that doesn't mean that I couldn't enjoy the competition.

Backgammon is quite different from chess. In chess, when you make a good move, you're rewarded with a better position. In backgammon, however, you're rewarded with better odds. Better odds means that there is still a small possibility of your opponent rolling a joker (i.e., an incredibly lucky roll) and turning the game around. With this space for luck, while there is no possibility for an average player to beat a world class player in chess, it is possible (though unlikely) for an average player to win against a world class backgammon player.

I've never met Kit Woolsey in person. He is both a world class backgammon player and a world class bridge player. He has written dozens of books on backgammon and on bridge. I'm familiar with some of his inventions in bridge, like the "Puppet Stayman" convention. I also read one of his backgammon books for calculating the odds for correct cube action, though it was over my head.

I was paired up against him at an online backgammon tournament. Once we met online to play our game, I knew this was a big moment because suddenly nearly one hundred people joined our table and started watching our match. Up to that point, I hadn't had even a single person watching my games; obviously, they were there to watch Woolsey's expected slaughter of an unknown player. The game started on time, and progressed normally, with nothing unusual happening. At one point the score was 3-3 with me surprisingly holding my own in a 7-point match. Meanwhile, I was skeptical that this equality would last long. A superior player like him was bound to play the better moves and sooner or later push me to the proverbial ropes. In a long game, where statistics would eventually catch up with me, and I would eventually make a mistake, I didn't stand a chance against him, but in a short game I could get lucky. Based on our rating differences, he would be a 66% favorite to win the match. That suggested that if I turned the cube when it seemed I had just over a 33% chance of winning, it would be a breakeven point for me. So, I decided to turn the cube early, which would be considered a mistake by analysis of more equal players. He had to accept of course: he had a slightly better position, he'd have the ownership of the cube, and he could turn it to four whenever he felt like. As the game progressed, it felt like the sword of Damocles was hanging over my neck. He did turn the cube to four eventually, offering it to me. I took some time to evaluate the situation. If I declined, which would be the correct move since he was in a better position, and he won the round, I would be trailing 3-5 in a 7-point game. I didn't think I could win four games against a player of his caliber before he won two more games. So, I accepted the cube and wished for the best even though he had a good lead on the board. With the cube at four in a 3-3 game of 7 points, whatever happened, this would be the last game of the match. After several lucky rolls in a row, I ended up winning, with those four cube points pushing me to 7. I cherish this win—achieved by embracing my limitations—to date.

* * *

At MDL, meanwhile, I was busy developing technical marketing material related to *MACCS-3D*, which was released in December 1989. It was the first commercially available 3D information management software on the market; other such software existed before *MACCS-3D*, but these programs were privately used in companies and were not publicly available for purchase.

For the technical documents I was working on to be provided to prospective clients, I needed some way to assess hitlists retrieved by various search queries: how good they were, based on their ability to stand for a set of compounds with desired biological activity. By analogy, if you are looking to buy a new car, you might use a search engine, input "new cars," and get a million possible results. Add limitations like top price, size, miles per gallon, and reliability, however, and your set of results is much reduced. Which combination of the above limitations give the best result? The best result is not necessarily the fewest cars to pick from, as you need to account for the quality of the cars and their suitability for your needs. And what about the quality to price ratio? The car buyer needs to be able to assess which search approach provides the most relevant results. Likewise, what the researchers needed was a way to evaluate the quality of the results from a pharmacophore search given specific sets of descriptors of the desired compounds.

To achieve this, I needed a useful metric. I consulted some of the people in the company who were well versed in mathematics, but they could not produce a satisfactory metric. In the end, I realized that I would have to develop one myself. Mathematics is not my forte, so I was struggling with where to start. The aim of chemical database searching is to be able to retrieve a hitlist with a substantial proportion of compounds with the desired properties. Following several searches that resulted in hitlists with different shapes and sizes, one would wonder which was the best result. Once determined, the search query that yielded the best result would be used as the best model.

Database search queries are mathematical models developed by incorporating the properties of a set of desired compounds that are missing in a set of undesired ones. For example, if we are trying to produce a predictive model that will differentiate biologically active compounds from those inactive ones for a specific target receptor enzyme (a specific lock), we can use a pharmacophore model, described above, as it tries to mimic the interaction between a receptor and a ligand that takes place in nature. Once a good pharmacophore model is available, scientists can use it to search databases of chemicals, and some of the new compounds retrieved with the model will be prospective potentially active new compounds. The better the predictive model, the more likely that the hitlist may have a useful new drug candidate.

So, I rolled up my sleeves and started working on developing a metric that would rank the pharmacophore models based on the quality of search results. Working with a colleague, Dr. Douglas R. Henry, it took us several years to come up with one. For the readers who may be interested, Appendix III details the stepwise development of the Goodness of Hitlist Score metric (GH-Score).

* * *

I was with MDL when I made my first trip to Japan. An American colleague who had lived there for a long time (in fact had his K-12 education there) gave me a crash course about Japan: how to greet each other, how to exchange business cards, meeting protocols, etc. He also introduced me to the unique cultural features of Japan: why consensus was so important for them, how one first should establish acquaintance and trust before talking business. I was intrigued by and could identify with these cultural aspects due to my Turkish heritage.

A large Japanese company sponsored this trip. Upon my arrival at the airport, a young guide and interpreter that the company had arranged greeted me. He escorted me to my hotel in Tokyo and left for home after agreeing to meet in the lobby the next morning at 7 a.m. He remained with me throughout my entire stay, picking me up each morning, taking me to my meetings at various locations. He dined with me and accompanied me through sometimes late-night dinner meetings and translated when needed. Towards the end of my visit, I asked him where he lived in Tokyo. I was surprised to learn that he lived outside Tokyo; he took public transportation with several changes to get back and forth via a two-hour one-way route. I calculated that he would need to get up at 4:00 -4:30 a.m. to get to my hotel by 7 a.m.; then he sometimes did not arrive back home until past midnight. This was the case for the entire week of my stay.

I found Tokyo intimidating on this first visit. It was crowded; the whole place was in constant motion with people moving in all directions around a city that seemed overly complex. Yet, remarkably, all the busses and trains arrived on time. I felt safe there regardless of the time of day. The fact that my introduction to Japan involved such exceptional hospitality made a permanent impression on me. Even today, Japan is my favorite country to visit. And I would not mind living there either.

* * *

During one of the American Chemical Society (ACS) national meetings on the East Coast, an important client visited our booth to check for the new *MACCS-3D* software. A scientist I knew from this company was hosting their VIPs and bringing them over to our booth. I said I would be happy to show them the software. However, my friend was not asking for a demonstration of the software but asking when Jason was going to be at the booth. I told him I had no idea, and he said he would tour the exposition area with the VIPs and check back at the booth in about an hour. The MDL account representative had insisted that they should receive the demo from Jason, an application scientist in the local office in New Jersey where the account representative also worked. Neither the account rep nor Jason was around. I had been asking about Jason's whereabouts, but no one seemed to know. The client came back a second time—this time he came alone—to ask if Jason had showed up. He said he wanted to make sure that he brought his VIPs when Jason was at the booth. Jason was still not around. So, he said he would bring them over to the booth in about 30 minutes, that he hoped that Jason would be there, and he left.

A little while later, a furious account representative came over and lashed out at me. She said, "How dare you send away my important clients not once, but twice." And continued "You should never speak to any of my clients again!" About five minutes later the director of marketing who oversaw the exposition asked why I would send off such important clients. I was dumbfounded.

Later, I saw that the client, with colleagues from his company's top echelons, receiving a demo from Jason. I looked over their shoulders and found it to be a poorly performed demo, mediocre at best. He was showing the client what happens when you push this button, and then what happens if you push the other button. Whereas when I do a demo, I do not directly show which buttons do what. Instead, I run through a research scenario and go through the proper use of the software tools to do the research. The recipient ends up seeing what happens when you push this or that button but in the context of a research scenario while performing a typical familiar task.

From my perspective, the account rep made a poor decision when she insisted her important client receive the demo from one person with whom she happened to have a good relationship. She also did not alert the booth personnel that a VIP visit was being scheduled. Not only did she risk alienating the VIPs by forcing them to wait for the requested individual, she also unknowingly settled for an inferior demo. I felt wronged, and the company could have lost an important client, but I did not know what to do about it. After returning to the office in California, I was considering calling the head of Sales to offer my perspective on the incident. Before I could call him, however, a company-wide announcement informed us that the account rep of concern was no longer with the company.

Much later, I developed a theory about why the account rep insisted that Jason do the demo. Shortly after I started working at MDL, as I walked to the office one day, I ran into Jason, who was visiting headquarters from our New Jersey office. As we walked together, he asked insistently how my interview had gone before I got the job offer. I told him that I was lucky because I thought I was not doing well until I responded to a question asking what the benefit of computer simulation was. I gave an example of my work in Alabama where I was designing rocket propellants. If I were doing actual experiments in a wet chemistry lab with these novel high energy compounds, I would be blowing up the lab half the time. Whereas we instead used computer simulations to sift through these dangerous compounds and could actually experiment on only those few promising candidates. The interviewers received this answer well, and I thought that was a decisive factor. So, I told Jason that the other finalist may have been better than me, but I got a lucky question with which I turned the odds in my favor. I was not sure if this was truly the case, but I was trying to be modest and show humility.

Eventually, I found out that the other finalist was Jason himself. So, after my modest rendering of my interview, he may have thought that he was actually the better candidate but somehow, unfairly, did not get my job. He may have shared this misconception with the account rep. If so, that may have explained why the account rep insisted on having Jason do the demo. Of course, I may be wrong.

In my experience, humility seems to be in decline in America. In today's cutthroat corporate environment, those who show modesty can quickly be eliminated. Conversely, those who shamelessly advertise themselves and exaggerate their skills seem to advance quickly and go far. This may also explain why I developed a fondness for Japan, where humility is still highly regarded.

\* \* \*

Zeynep got a job as a programmer analyst at a company in San Bruno, which was across the San Francisco Bay, about an hour away. We decided to move to San Bruno to shorten her commute. I would now have to cross the San Mateo Bay Bridge for my commute. This was around 1990, a year after the big Loma Prieta earthquake, when a part of the Bay Bridge had collapsed and the traffic on the San Mateo bridge, which I would have to take, had practically doubled. We found an apartment at the top of a hill in San Bruno, right on top of the San Andreas Fault. A lot of houses (but not ours) were advertising that their property was "below the fog line". I didn't know what it meant at that time. I found out soon enough.

My daughter, Sibel, was born in Redwood City on Mother's Day in 1990. She was breached, and regardless of how many times the doctor tried to correct her position, she would flip back to the breach position as if she were doing this deliberately. Was this an indication of her personality? Would she be a stubborn, independent person, who always must have her own way? In the end, the doctors gave up, and Sibel was born through C-section. We were now a family of four and settled into a routine.

As we approached the middle of summer, a dense fog would settle in. It was not a stationary fog, though; it was in motion, a rolling cloud of sorts. We could see this fog move from the ocean to inland. When it was dense, its movement was so distinct that I felt if I opened the front door and the back balcony door, the fog would go right through our apartment. I was so intrigued with this natural phenomenon that I wanted to attach an identity to it and so decided to call it "George." A typical family comment would be something like "George is thick and fast-moving today."

Friends who were visiting us from San Jose would bring their winter clothing with them because it could be some ten to fifteen degrees colder than San Jose. The fact that we almost lived inside the clouds quickly got stale. You could go quarter of a mile in any direction, and it would be bright and sunny. Yet in our neighborhood, it would be hazy and gloomy. Now I appreciated the ads for houses noting that they were below the fog line. In later years, whenever we'd see a rolling cloud coming down a hill in that area, we'd salute George. I later learned that San Franciscans called it Karl. So, it seems, I was not the first-person giving names to low rolling clouds.

* * *

An account rep invited me to a meeting at a French multinational pharmaceutical company that had just gone through a large merger. He wanted me to show them the latest version of our software and to give a presentation on its scientific merits. In the audience, in addition to about ten scientists from the host company, was another scientist who had traveled from Switzerland and was from the other company in the just-completed merger. I did not know the history, but this person was a supporter of a competitor product. I remembered seeing a poster co-authored by him where the authors presented some research data and interpreted it in what I thought was a biased manner to support their favored product. That same data was also in my presentation, but I had a different interpretation of it. He got upset and became hostile, almost implying that I was lying. I did not know how to respond to that. If I was alone and representing only myself, I would debate the issue. But I was there standing for my company and at the invitation of another client. What a conundrum! I could not continue arguing with him in the presence of my host. So I swallowed my pride, de-escalated the situation, and completed my presentation. But the experience had a lasting mark on me. I had never felt so humiliated before. I came to realize that some people perceived me as a salesperson rather than a scientist. In their view, my company was a "vendor," and I was out there to support a sale, not advocate for genuine science.

I should not have allowed these slights to influence me. It was time for me to develop a thicker skin. It would take some time, but I would get to the point of being able to let such situations wash off me, prioritizing more important things in life.

* * *

Twice a week, a group of us would go to the San Leandro Marina to play ultimate frisbee during our lunch break. The game resembles football without body contact. An offensive player tosses a frisbee much like a quarterback throws a football, and a wide receiver tries to catch it, of course competing with the defensive catchers. Unlike in football, you cannot run when you have the frisbee but must toss it to another player before being able to run again. You advance the position by passing the frisbee from player to player, and someone has to catch the frisbee in the end zone to score.

With all the running back and forth and jumping to catch or block the frisbee, the sport is extremely cardiovascular. At each break, most of us would be desperate to catch our breath. Ultimate frisbee became my major physical activity. I believe I achieved my peak physical condition during these times. So much so that when I had a lingering cold bothering me and eventually went to the doctor, he said something like, "How could you possibly be here? You should not have been able to even get out of bed in this condition." I had pneumonia. Because I was in such good physical condition, I hadn't realized how much my body was fighting the infection. He prescribed an antibiotic, and when I woke up the next morning, I felt so great that I thought, this must be how it is to be born again.

* * *

Hülya and Kemal had their daughter Deniz with them for one of their visits. We explored the sights in San Francisco, but because the kids were getting bored, we decided to go to Disneyworld in Los Angeles for a couple of days. Deniz at about seven years old and Kurt at five joined us for the trip. Zeynep couldn't come because of her job and stayed in San Francisco with two-year-old Sibel. Deniz and Kurt enjoyed both Disneyworld and the pool at the hotel where we stayed. At one point, Kurt's bathing suit got loose and dropped as he played in the pool. As he was frantically trying to pull it up, he noticed Deniz watching him with wide eyes. He said, "Your stay here is short, but we ended up knowing each other real fast." Kurt was already witty as a kid, and still is as an adult.

* * *

Meanwhile, my marriage wasn't going well. Zeynep and I had our differences, but more importantly, we couldn't seem to communicate with each other. We continued to have different recollections of the same events and could not reconcile. I also remember overhearing a conversation Zeynep had with some Turkish friends. When they asked, "Should we check with Osman first," she said, "I don't care what he thinks." A multitude of such little things was starting to add up. We tried couples counseling. After a few sessions, Zeynep started to have arguments with the therapist, too. She didn't trust the process and wanted to bring a tape recorder to our sessions. So it didn't work. We agreed to file for divorce.

Kurt was six years old, and Sibel was three. I moved out of our apartment in San Bruno to an apartment in San Leandro across the Bay, walking distance from MDL. Sibel would stay with Zeynep, and Kurt would stay with me. During the weekends, the kids would come together alternating with me or with Zeynep.

San Leandro boasted a golf course within walking distance of my place. Alone during the weekends when the kids were with Zeynep, I started to take some lessons, acquired a set of clubs, and began to play golf seriously. This would be my main outdoor activity for many years. I also acquired my first PC and the software called *Street Smart* to start learning Wall Street investment strategies. I put aside $10,000 as play money and started experimenting with different investment schemes. This became my main hobby. I spent an hour or more every night studying the market. I would use these investment strategies for the rest of my life.

The kids weren't happy being separated from each other, and when Kurt started preschool, he wasn't doing well. During my business trips, Zeynep would drive Kurt to his school, unfortunately far away from her residence. It was tough going for the kids, and it was tough going for Zeynep as well.

Our family friends were gently probing, feeling out whether Zeynep and I could make up and come together again. We were part of a small Turkish community which would meet socially once a month or so. Our Turkish friends were all married with small children, so these gatherings were especially good for the kids. Once, the host set up a game, like the *Newlywed Game* TV show, where couples compete to answer questions related to their partners (in their absence) to see which couple knows each other the best. All the couples were married, and they had been together for considerable amounts of time. We were the only separated couple but nevertheless we won. They pushed this as further evidence that we knew each other so well that we should get back together. I wondered if they faked their own answers so that we would win.

The arrival of Kurt's report card, which was sub-par, brought us to the tipping point and helped us decide to get back together, toughing it out until the kids were old enough to handle the separation. We leased a house in Fremont and moved in. The family was, once again, together under one roof. After our first year in Fremont, we decided to buy a nearby house and settle down—the first home we owned in the US.

\* \* \*

I had an anxious call from an MDL account representative saying that a newly founded pharmaceutical company, Vertex, was considering making a large investment in our software systems, but they had several technical questions that he could not answer. He said this was an important opportunity and could I please call Dr. Mark Murcko over at Vertex to address his questions. As a brand-new company, Vertex had a big budget for their computer-aided drug design group. I called and was directed to Dr. Murcko's voicemail. I told him who I was, gave my number, and told him that I would be happy to address any questions he might have about our software systems. I did not hear back from him right away, but I got a call from the account representative a little later. He was overly excited. He said I was a hero; he said that Vertex bought a large installation of our software systems and whatever I had done must have worked. I said I had not done anything, but he would not listen, telling everyone that I helped him make this big sale. So, I was credited for something I had not done and was a hero (despite my consistent objections) for about half a day. Eventually, the truth came out. Vertex had as one of its goals to acquire all available recent technology to help them design new drugs. It turned out that they were buying tools from all companies, including our competitors. I was quite relieved to have the burden of unwarranted credit lifted off my shoulders.

\* \* \*

Kurt started doing well in school, a big relief for us, validating our decision to come together, albeit temporarily. The school had a gifted and talented education (GATE) program that we thought Kurt should participate in. He would have to take an exam and undergo an evaluation first. One day, unbeknownst to us, Kurt was summoned out of his class to the principal's office for this evaluation and exam. Kurt didn't know what was happening, and he was frightened and nervous. Had he done something wrong? In this scary environment, he was subjected to the IQ test as well. Despite his anxiety, the test results left no question of where he belonged; Kurt continued his elementary education within GATE.

Like me, Kurt was into books. He would read them out loud and, at a certain point, I would turn the book upside down, and he would continue reading aloud without skipping a beat. I never understood how he read the words seeing them upside down. His passion for reading continued into adulthood. He would finish reading a book quickly with full comprehension of its contents, which made me envious. I liked reading too, but in the process, I would soon start daydreaming and would end up having to go back to read again to understand the bits that I missed. Kurt was also a peacemaker. Calm, collected, he approached and helped his friends with their problems all the time. Consequently, he was popular.

* * *

We had hired a new product manager who also reported to my boss. We organized a welcome treat at a coffee place to introduce him to the group in a relaxed, fun meeting. We were joking around and having fun. At one point, from a little distance, I overheard him talking about me to my boss's boss, and I heard him say "and this must be the class clown." He followed that with some racist remarks. My boss's boss was visibly uncomfortable with the exchange and was trying to hush him down. I was shocked. He didn't even know who I was. So, I had a bad start with this new hot shot. It turned out that he could talk the talk but could not walk the walk.

One day, I was rushing to one of my product team meetings, and he started to tag along. I asked what he wanted and said that I was in a hurry to get to my meeting. He wanted to come to my meeting with me. The developers on his product team, frustrated with the way he handled his team meetings, had sent him to attend some of my team meetings so that he could learn how to run a meeting from me.

I had designed my meetings to be efficient. I set up the agenda and stuck to it, diligently taking notes, especially for action requests. I would list all the action requests at the end of the meeting and get approval from the people having to carry out the actions. And after the meeting, when I distributed the meeting minutes, at the top of the report was those actions that had not yet been completed, followed by the action requests for the following week. Since the minutes went to all the upper management, nobody wanted to stay on the top list more than a few weeks. So, I never had to chase people down to get them to do what they had promised to do. They were motivated to close the action so that they could get off the top list.

The new product manager was struggling at the company, and frequently he would call my boss to tell him that he was working from home that day. My boss was nice enough to allow for that without questioning. In one of those working-from-home days, apparently, he traveled to another city for a job interview. A short while later he left the company.

* * *

I was involved with the ACS Short Courses in *Computational Chemistry* (a name later changed to *Computer-Aided Drug Design*). These short courses lasted the two days just before the technical program began at ACS national meetings. Tens of thousands of chemists from all around the world attended, and some arrived early to take advantage of the meeting to attend the short courses. ACS offered about two dozen of these courses. In 1990, by invitation from Dr. J. Phillip Bowen, the organizer of the short course, I joined the faculty of this short course series. This short course that several other scientists and I contributed to represented one of the longest running ACS short courses, continuing for nearly two decades until 2009. I taught it for 19 years. The full-length version of this course had a lab component as well, excluded from the two-day course due to time constraints. In addition to the short course attached to ACS National meetings, we held the full four-day course with its hands-on lab sessions at one of the sponsoring universities at some other scheduled time. Most of the students were from industry, some at the management level, trying to understand the new emerging technologies that their companies were getting involved with. With these ACS courses, Phil Bowen and I started and evolved a long-lasting friendship.

* * *

One spring, after a few years with the company, I was invited to meet with a Dr. Robin Breckenridge from the major multinational company Roche in Switzerland. According to the account representative, he was skeptical and critical of our recent technology and had some tough questions. He was also influential not only within his company, but also on the European scientific scene. The account rep asked me to give a presentation with the latest scientific updates to the software. I was happy to do so, of course, and put together a nice presentation that I believed covered all key issues that a critical scientist might have. It started well, but his skepticism was clear. He often interrupted me with some deep questions. At a certain point, I moved to the white board and spent the next forty-five minutes addressing all his questions. I was not able to go back to my prepared presentation. After I returned to the US, the account rep called me to say that his client was satisfied with our meeting, and that this was the first time he had ever supplied positive feedback.

This experience was educational for me. However great your presentation may be, it is more important to listen to your audience and adopt your delivery to address their needs. You should be willing to abandon your presentation entirely, if necessary, to communicate successfully. This was also a validation for me, personally. One can only achieve this higher level of communication if you first recognize the needs but also then have the knowledge to answer the problematic questions. I felt like I was coming into my own, career wise. It seemed I had grown quite a bit since my start at MDL. I had gathered a high level of respect in the company. I was getting fewer insults and a lot more accolades.

I had good support from the Corporate Communications staff for my activities. Even though my English language skills had significantly improved, I still needed help with material I developed for external use. A friend, Lise Dumont, was particularly supportive and we worked well together. Her contributions to the papers were significant and beyond editorial support, so I felt she should be listed as a coauthor to a few of the documents,[13] and one peer-reviewed scientific paper as well.[14] As someone with only a bachelor's degree in science, she recently indicated that she is grateful for the nod and proud of these scientific publications to this day.

Towards the end of my tenure at MDL, *MACCS-3D* was being demoted because it did not generate the expected revenues. Management was considering moving some of the developers of *MACCS-3D* to some other projects. I tried to delay that; I made one last plea to the chief executive officer (CEO), Steven Goldby, and his vice presidents to keep the team together a little longer, arguing that new technologies take some time to be adopted. After the meeting, the director of Development was happy and thought that I saved the day. I was not so sure.

The writing was on the wall. Bringing 3D into a world that was firmly established in two dimensions was like rowing against the current—and I was getting tired of the effort. So, when I got signals from Accelrys about a possible position, I was open to the idea. At least Accelrys was a company firmly established in 3D, and I would be rowing with the stream there. When I accepted the position at Accelrys, people at MDL were understanding and acknowledged that this was a good move for me.

Following my several days of debriefing, the goodbye luncheon, and parting praises, my boss walked me to the door for the final time and told me about some of the conversations about me they had had at their upper-level meetings. For instance, the CEO was complaining about some people who would not finish projects and would keep tweaking things trying to perfect them. He was saying "Why can't they be just like Osman. Get the project completed, bring it to a close, and then move on to another project." Naturally, hearing this felt good.

# CHAPTER 7

# At Accelrys

*San Diego, California, 1996-2005*

Accelrys recruited me from MDL in 1996 to a Senior Product Manager position for their chemistry products. One of the software products I would manage was *Catalyst*. Compared to *MACCS-3D*, *Catalyst* had more functionality and capability and represented the next generation of pharmacophore modeling; modern, powerful, and effective. Possibly, it was one of the reasons *MACCS-3D* sales at MDL were suffering. Accelrys had acquired the company that had developed *Catalyst* (that company's only product).

Accelrys was not going to integrate *Catalyst* into any of its existing platforms immediately and would maintain it as a standalone product. This approach was probably a reason I was selected for my role. *Catalyst* was complex, and since it was not to be part of one of Accelrys' existing platforms, not many people could manage it. The person who was managing it then, Dr. Scott Kahn (who came to Accelrys with the *Catalyst* acquisition), was due for promotion but, apparently, did not want to move on until he found someone to take over managing *Catalyst*. He was to become my boss with his promotion to vice president of Marketing, and he wanted to hire someone who could champion this emerging technology. He knew that I had been involved with the release of the first commercial 3D-search software at MDL. We had met at scientific meetings and conferences several times. Because conference organizers typically combine related presentations together in the same session, Scott and I presented back-to-back several times, sometimes as competitors, and sometimes as colleagues. So it wasn't surprising that he thought I would be a good person to take over the management of *Catalyst*.

When I flew out to San Diego for my interview, the gate agent told me that my seat had been upgraded to first class. Surprised, I went in and settled in my seat. A few minutes later, Scott sat down, right next to me. He was flying to San Diego as well and had arranged our adjacent seats. He and I developed an excellent relationship over many years. He was a supportive manager. Slightly balding and wearing metal-rimmed glasses, at about six feet, two inches tall he made a big presence, and he was a force to be reckoned with. Today, when I look back, I realize I was lucky to have him as my mentor and manager. He not only had superior technical knowledge but was also able to navigate corporate politics well. I appreciated his support whenever I felt stuck.

For example, one night I was working on a demonstration of a prototype software application for our Japan Users' Group Meeting, and I was stuck. The system not working. It was 9 p.m. already and I was scheduled to fly out early the next morning. I was ready to give up and called Scott at his home as a last resort. Amazingly, he instructed me over the phone, step by step, on how to get the prototype working and interacting with the system. An hour later, I was able to develop a narrow research scenario that I could use to demonstrate the future possibilities of this prototype application. It was a narrow scenario so that if I veered slightly from the planned path, the whole thing would collapse. But I was intent on demonstrating the prototype: a picture is worth a thousand words. With Scott's help I now had something to show, and the demo in Japan was successful.

I always remembered this incident as demonstrating how supportive Scott was, helping me out late at night from home. Interestingly, his perspective on the incident was that I would not give up and was working hard, late at night, to get things done before a critical meeting, and he appreciated that. Scott eventually became the Chief Scientific Officer at Accelrys, and when the company was failing and the turn-around specialists took over the management of the company, he (wisely) jumped ship and swiftly found another job as Chief Information Officer at Illumina, Inc.

Accelrys gave me a relocation package for my move to San Diego. The company moved our household goods and two cars to San Diego and stored all but what we needed until we purchased our new home there. They hired professionals to help with the sale of our house in Fremont and helped buy our new house in San Diego once we chose it. Until then, they accommodated us in a fully furnished corporate apartment. Accelrys made the relocation process as painless as possible for me so that I could focus and be productive with my work.

We did our research and identified the neighborhood where we wanted to settle. We would buy a house in the San Diego neighborhood where the public schools had the highest rating. The house values were at a premium in that area, but Zeynep and I agreed that we would always prioritize the kids' needs.

Our new house in the Del Mar Heights area, at the north end of San Diego, was close to a top-ranked public high school. Since he was still too young for high school, we registered Kurt for the Skyline School at Solano Beach.

A month later, when Zeynep and I were walking together to a school activity, one of the parents approached us and said, "It's okay, my son and Kurt get along fine, and they're good friends again." We had no idea what she was talking about.

We later learned that Kurt had been involved in confrontation with her kid, and they had both received detention time. Kurt had never mentioned this to us, probably because he was embarrassed. When we talked to the principle and the teacher who had witnessed the event and learned that Kurt had been trying to defend himself, we were dissatisfied with their response and upset about what we felt was an unbalanced reprimand.

Shortly after, we moved Kurt to a private Montessori school. He seemed to blame himself for the change and took some time to adopt to the new environment. Eventually, he settled in and did well in school, and we were all happy.

When Sibel came to school age, we didn't even consider public school for her and had her start at Kurt's Montessori school. She did well and pulled all A's, but she wasn't happy there. After she finished the second grade, Sibel took a required standard national test. As a result, some magnet schools invited her to transfer in.

San Diego offered a program called "seminar" for children who scored above 99% in this national exam. The top "sub-percentile" was invited to attend this special program with high educational standards. We asked a couple of her teachers at the Montessori school for advice, and they discouraged the transfer. Her teacher said that the kids in these schools had a lot of homework and were under a lot of pressure. Despite this discouragement, Zeynep insisted that we transfer Sibel to one of the magnet schools that was some twelve miles from our home, and I agreed.

This was a good decision. Sibel was happy, developed good study habits, and received an excellent education. I was impressed to see that the students were learning "combinations" and "permutations" in elementary school. I had first been exposed to this level of math in college. More importantly, Sibel fit in. Among kids like herself, she felt normal. These creative kids showed their stuff when her friends spent weekends at our house. One weekend, Sibel, and one of her friends visiting, decided to make a movie with a single video recorder. Sibel would speak to the camera, then turn to her right as if there were someone right next to her and say, "don't you agree?" Then the next shot would start with her friend looking left and saying that she agreed, and then she turned to the camera and continued. This way they gave the impression that they had been side by side when shooting the scenes, even though one of them was always running the camera.

They also used our yellow Lab, Goldie, in their movies. When they decided to add a second doggie character to a movie, they put a red bandana on Goldie to distinguish her from her first character. By the end of the weekend, they would typically have produced a short movie. Sibel regularly preoccupied herself with such projects.

One day at school, Sibel was summoned into the administrator's office during a physical education class. The executive assistant to the principal was having a hard time with her computer and someone suggested Sibel take a look at it. It so happened that a few weeks earlier I had showed her how to navigate computer menus using Alt, Tab, and arrow keys in case the mouse didn't work. Since that happened to be the problem with this person's computer—the mouse didn't work— Sibel was able to help by expertly navigating the menus from the keyboard to reboot the system. The reboot revived the mouse so, within three minutes, to the amazement of the people watching, nine-years-old Sibel had solved the problem.

While Sibel was receiving a great education, Zeynep had to drive her the twelve miles to and from school every day, a sacrifice I very much appreciated. With this strong start, Sibel too progressed smoothly through San Diego's educational system.

* * *

In June 1998, I got a call from my sister, Mine, in Turkey that my father had had another heart attack when the family was visiting Istanbul, and he was hospitalized. His condition was serious. I was on the next flight to Istanbul. My cousins met me at the airport. While we were driving to my cousin's home, I asked if we could stop by the hospital so that I could see my father. But he had passed that morning. Sadly, I was too late.

The whole family gathered in my aunt's home, including people whom I hadn't seen for many years, and a few distant relatives I didn't know at all. Even though my father was secular, we prayed. Many people were going in and out giving condolences to Mom, my sister and me. A lot of thoughts and conversations around my father's accomplishments. Reminiscences about his personality, jokes, and adventures. I was dazed; I wasn't hearing much of the conversations.

We honored several ritualistic traditions, and finally held the funeral. We buried him next to my grandfather's grave in a spot for which we already had the deed. My mother let us know she was expecting to be buried there when her time came, even though she lived in Ankara. Surrounded by old trees and well-maintained flora, it was a beautiful and peaceful cemetery, a great final resting place.

My grandfather had immigrated from Thessaloniki Greece as part of an exchange of ethnic Turks and Greeks after World War I. This cemetery was founded after the migrations, and the majority of the deeds were owned by those who had emigrated from Greece, just as my ancestors had. After the funeral, we all returned to Ankara where my sister, Mine handled the many necessary bureaucratic procedures. After a few more days of reflection, I returned to San Diego.

* * *

Meanwhile, it had been five years since we had received our Green Cards, so we were eligible to apply for citizenship. US citizenship was important to me because I still struggled when organizing my visas on international business trips. Following my father's passing, I was in no mood for such bureaucracy and decided to hire a lawyer to manage the citizenship application. When I called an attorney specialized in immigration, the first question he asked was "What's wrong?" Sensing my hesitancy, he continued, "What is the problem we need to deal with to get you citizenship?" I said, "Nothing, no problem at all." Then continued, "It has been five years since we received our green cards, and we want to apply for citizenship." He said, "Just go to the government web site and fill out the application form." So that's what I did.

We each took and passed our citizenship test and then received a date for the citizenship ceremony. I was so busy at work that I didn't have much time to even think about it. When the day came, we went to the site of the ceremony. It was a large theatre with about five hundred people in it. People gave talks and at one point, a speaker started naming the countries represented in the room and asking people from those countries to stand up. When Turkey was called, only Zeynep and I stood up. When Mexico was called, practically everybody in the room stood up.

I know that for many people this ceremony is important and memorable. But for me it was anticlimactic. I was thinking about the many things going on at work during the ceremony. Once we received the naturalization document, though, I immediately applied for a US passport. Ever since, my international travels have been relatively straightforward.

* * *

I made my first father-son trip with Kurt one weekend when he was ten years old. We made a two-and-a-half-hour drive from San Diego to a chess tournament in Los Angeles and checked in to the hotel where the tournament was held. Kurt had learned how to play chess when he was five and did okay for a while but never took it seriously. This tournament had a section for the kids, and I thought he might gain some experience playing in a competitive environment and, perhaps, rekindle his interest in chess. Kurt didn't do so well in his section, but we had a fun time together. And, of course, for Kurt, hanging out with Dad, staying in a hotel, dining out, playing in the pool, was all a lot of fun.

A unique exhibition was headed towards the US in 2001: "Palace of Gold and Light: Treasures from the Topkapi, Istanbul." It would be exhibited at three sites: in Washington, DC; Fort Lauderdale, Florida; and, from July 14 to September 24, at the San Diego Museum of Art. The Turkish consulate in Los Angeles was encouraging Turkish citizens living in Southern California to help support the event. Since San Diego was our city, Zeynep decided to volunteer to help with fund raising and promotion. For one event, Zeynep opened our house to the participants.

A group of high-school students visiting from Turkey performed folk dances in our large back yard. About one hundred people overall enjoyed the entertainment along with talks and food, including hors d'oeuvres and a BBQ. Zeynep was busy during the reception. I was also working hard and assisting with the logistics but was not hosting the event. This was Zeynep's role, and I decided to take a back seat. My being invisible allowed me to hear some of the respected(!) members of the Los Angeles Turkish community making some condescending remarks about Zeynep. I wondered what to do. Should I confront them and risk making a scene? If I didn't, how would I convey this to Zeynep? We were not communicating well with each other at the time, and I didn't think she would believe me. In the end, I decided not to mention it to Zeynep.

While I was walking around in the house and collecting trash, a woman came over and started talking with me. When she realized I was Zeynep's husband she said, "Oh, so this is your house?" My response came out without me even thinking. "No," I said. "I am paying for most of it, but this is not my house." I was surprised at my own words. It was the first time I realized that I didn't feel I belonged in my own house.

This was one of the several events for fund raising in Southern California but the only one in San Diego, and it was a success. The exhibition opened in July and was well attended, providing a unique opportunity for locals and San Diego tourists to learn about the life-styles of Ottoman Sultans. Normally, one would have to travel to Turkey and visit the Topkapi Palace to see these treasures.

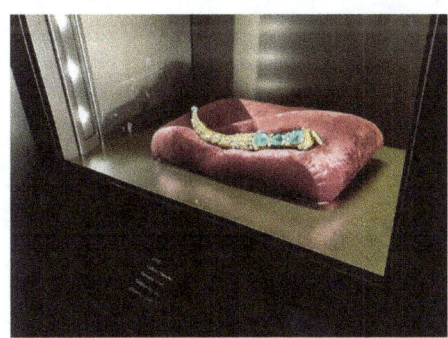

The Topkapi Dagger was the subject of the 1964 movie "Topkapi," in which a gang attempted to steal it.

The exhibition was a success, and the Los Angeles consulate organized a reception to recognize some of the volunteers, including Zeynep. The recognitions included an award. She asked me if I could go with her. I was stuck. I really didn't want to take the two-hour drive, one way, with her and then face what I perceived as the hypocrisy and superficiality of the people at the reception. So I declined, assuming she would make the trip on her own as she had with her previous engagements with the LA folk. She decided not to go without me. I later realized I was wrong. We were still married, and I should have stood by my wife during this event. I have regretted my selfish response ever since.

\* \* \*

Sometime after I became proficient with the *Catalyst* system, I was considered an expert in this area, and the sales force would use me as the *big gun* whenever a prospect needed some scientific persuasion. My job required me to travel globally about ten percent of the time. One of my favorite destinations was Japan. I admired the cultural aspects of the country (like honoring one's word and trust, respecting elders, humility, loyalty). With my Turkish origins, I could identify with these values. I would typically visit Japan twice a year, mostly for our annual Japan Users' Group Meetings, some speaking engagements at conferences, or to meet with clients and prospects when requested by the account representatives.

Getting ready for one of these trips to Japan, I got a phone call from a friend, Dr. Jim Kaminski, who worked at Schering-Plough Corporation, a pharmaceutical company. I was not surprised by his call since he was speaking at the same meeting, and he might have some questions about it. Perhaps he wanted to schedule a dinner with me during the conference. Instead, he was calling with incredibly sad news. He told me that he had recently been diagnosed with late-stage pancreatic cancer and had at once started a chemotherapy regimen.

I was devastated. He was a good scientist with many years of productive and creative work in front of him. And at this relatively young age, he was now fighting for his life. I could not talk. "My doctor," he continued, "won't allow me to travel to Japan. My presentation is complete, and I wanted to ask you if you could deliver it on my behalf."

"I would be honored to do that, of course," I told him, and he sent me his presentation which explored how his company was able to make new discoveries using the pharmacophore modeling technology. The compounds that were displayed in his presentation were not proprietary, in fact, they had been published recently.[15] I was familiar with his paper since I had read it already as a success story and validation for this recent technology that I was championing. We started having phone meetings every several days to go through his presentation so that I would understand and learn the contents thoroughly, not only enough to deliver the presentation accurately, but also to be able to address questions from the audience after. Depending on how close our phone meeting was to his most recent chemotherapy session, I could feel how much pain Jim was enduring from the way he talked. Talking with him was difficult for me, but once we concentrated on science, it got easier.

Finally, the important day came in Japan. I got up to the podium to introduce Jim's talk and explained that Dr. Kaminski apologized for not being able to make the meeting personally due to a last-minute family emergency. Nobody knew that he was fighting for his life. Since I had been thoroughly coached by my friend, I gave a good presentation. At the end of the meeting, a survey for the participants asked how they would rank the presentations. Two presentations were singled out, receiving the highest votes. The top one was, as expected, Jim's talk, and the second one was my own talk on the latest developments in the pharmacophore technology. Jim passed away several months later.

* * *

ACS National Meetings were important for the two software companies that I had worked for, MDL (1989-1996) and Accelrys (1996-2005). Software companies tend to get numerous sales leads at these meetings since the prospects could see the tools demonstrated by experts in familiar contexts. We would usually opt for a large booth in a prominent location on the exposition floor, for instance, right across from the main entrance. The twenty to thirty thousand attendees made the ACS National meetings the largest in the chemistry field. Representatives from the medical, biological, and biotechnology fields also participated.

While the main goal of our ACS participation was marketing and sales, I thought our involvement with the technical program would be beneficial as well. The technical program was the main objective of these meetings, bringing together scientists from around the world to deliver talks on the latest developments in their respective areas at numerous symposia organized throughout the week. At any given point, several dozen different lectures might be running in parallel in different divisions. The exposition, on the other hand, was optional for the participants. At their booths, several hundred or so vendor companies would display their solutions for problems attendees faced in their work.

By taking part in the technical program, we could talk science with our clients and prospects without the obscuring sales talk that they would normally receive on the exposition floor. Scientists at Accelrys would normally present occasional papers in the relevant symposia as new products were developed, but I wanted to take this concept further. Our extended involvement would be multi-faceted: performing scientific research, publishing in scientific journals (preferably co-authored with some of our clients) and giving scientific presentations at various relevant symposia at ACS. I thus incorporated submitting for publication peer-reviewed scientific articles into the annual objectives of my product managers. To my knowledge this was unique to my group. While this would be additional work for them, they appreciated the opportunity to enhance their *curricula vitae* that this presented. The effort both increased their value for the company and their standing in the industry—as well as their scientific cachet—for future job opportunities.

In addition, I thought it was important for me to be involved with the leadership of various divisions of ACS. The information management software systems that we were involved with made the Chemical Information Division the most relevant for us.

After first attending the talks in the Division of Chemical Information at a meeting, I realized that the target audience seemed primarily to be librarians. These librarians are typically employed at academic institutions, though large, research-based chemical and pharmaceutical companies have their own specialized libraries. My vision for chemical information encompassed a wider coverage comprising scientific information management and applications. I approached one of the leaders of the division and asked him why the symposia in the technical program were restricted only to topics relevant to librarians or chemical databases but did not cover the scientific use of these databases. His response was that the Division of Computers in Chemistry was more appropriate for such topics.

I was not satisfied with his answer and disagreed with it. Unhappy with this situation, I expressed my opinion to my colleagues. Then I realized that I had no right to complain since I had not made any effort to deal with the situation myself. Considering that my job required me to take part in future ACS meeting expositions anyway, I should be able to take a more active role in the technical program of the Division of Chemical Information by managing my time effectively during future meetings.

The Division committees typically met a day before the start of the ACS technical program, so for the next ACS meeting, I traveled to the site a day early and attended the Division of Chemical Information, Program Committee meeting. I volunteered to organize a symposium for each of the meetings for the next three years (the following six ACS meetings). I had named six topics in the area of scientific information management and proposed these as symposium titles. I ended up being a volunteer participating in the Program Committee from 1998-2001 and then joining as an associate program chair from 2001-2003 before becoming program chair from 2003-2004. For years I organized at least one scientific symposium for the Division of Chemical Information at each of the ACS National Meetings. Appendix IV lists the titles of these symposia.

The ACS Chemical Information Division's technical program evolved with my contributions, enriched to include new topics like algorithms, applications, research, and inventions. Due to the resulting overlap with the Division of Computers in Chemistry, we started co-sponsoring each other's programs so that our symposia would be advertised in both division's programs. As soon as my term as the program chair ended, I was nominated and elected for the chair position, which was another three-year commitment as chair-elect in the first year, chair in the next, and past chair in the final year. Hence, I was heavily involved in the leadership of the Division for about a decade. During this time, the Division of Chemical Information had become diverse and vibrant with growing participation and substantial visibility. Two of the symposia that I had organized made it to the cover of the ACS publication *Chemical & Engineering News*.[16],[17] Since ACS has more than 30 technical divisions and several subdivisions, this was a welcome honor.

\* \* \*

San Diego's Torrey Pines High School was a short walk from our home, one of the criteria we used when we were house hunting. The school had nearly four thousand students, so it was effectively the scale of a college, and had a great reputation in the region. Kurt joined the basketball team his freshman year there, with rigorous practices every night after school. He was good enough to be on the team, but not good enough to be a starter and get a lot of court time. He realized that he didn't have the skills to be competitive in basketball. Regardless, he did not bail out as most of his friends did, and remained in the program, enduring the very demanding practice schedule until the end of his first year. Then he quit the basketball team.

When Sibel started at Torrey Pines High School, Kurt was in his senior year and a member of the speech and debate team. Sibel had missed the deadline to sign up herself, but Zeynep met with the coach and convinced her to add Sibel to the team. There she could have some face time with the big brother she practically worshipped. In one of the competitions, Kurt and his partner were eliminated from the tournament, while Sibel and her partner qualified for the State finals. Kurt handled this interesting development well.

Some years later, when Kurt was receiving his Eagle Scout badge, he wrote an essay about how he felt being one-upped by his little sister. His scout master was impressed with Kurt's reflections and told us that he was mature for his age. Indeed, Kurt was the peacemaker in the family and was the best big brother a younger sibling could hope for.

\* \* \*

On one of my trips to Japan, I was invited to a private meeting with a pharmaceutical company's chemistry group who were using our software systems. Usually, an account rep and some technical personnel from our Japan subsidiary would accompany me, so this request for a private meeting was unusual. When I arrived, my host greeted me and quickly whisked me off to a large meeting room with a workstation in the middle of a table, connected to a large-screen display. They had me, the software's guru, sitting in front of the workstation with a dozen or so scientists standing in a semi-circle behind me.

They were worried that their lead compounds in a particular project might fall under a recent patent application by a competitor in the US. I was familiar with the patent application involving a pharmacophore model. The patent was published but had not yet been issued. It was likely that it would not be issued any time soon since mathematical models were not patentable at that time. Scientists in the company were able to duplicate the model using the details published in the patent document. They wanted me to check if their compounds were within the domain of the model. I checked each one of their compounds under consideration. I performed a flexible, three-dimensional fitting of each compound onto the pharmacophore model. They all matched, meaning that if the patent were issued, these compounds would end up being worthless, falling under the patent protection of the competitor company.

I suspected they had already given up on those compounds and wanted a final validation from me. Otherwise, I would have been re-quired to sign pages of nondisclosure documents before they would let me see their compounds. Nevertheless, I was honored by the trust they had bestowed upon me.

In one of my later trips to Japan, a new account representative wanted me to visit a client who had several technical questions about the technology. This was the first time I was meeting with both this new account rep and the client. The client must have been particularly important to the account rep. He was nervous. Throughout the drive he coached me on how to interact with the client, what to do and what not to do. I listened patiently and promised to be on my best behavior. We arrived and were led to a large conference room, with about a dozen scientists already seated around the table. Less than a minute after I sat down, before I even opened my briefcase, one of the scientists came over with a hard copy of one of my recent review papers, wanting me to autograph it. With the ice broken, we had a cordial, pleasant, and mutually beneficial meeting.

Meanwhile, the GH-Score I had developed with Dr. Henry to rate the value of search hitlists was getting some attention. We needed to publish it. So, we worked on two papers. The first one laid out the theory that showed the derivation of the equation and was coauthored by me and Dr. Doug Henry; the second one was an applications paper coauthored by myself and Dr. Marvin Waldman. It took several months to complete the papers and finally to get them sent to the *Journal of Chemical Information and Computer Science.*

About another few months later Marvin asked what had happened with the papers. I checked with the editor. He was apologetic and said he had misplaced them and would send them out for peer review at once. I was disappointed at the delay. Then the journal seemed to have rushed the review process since just about a month later, I got the reviewers' comments, one of them negative. Today I don't remember the particulars of the objections, but I remember being upset that the reviewer did not understand our premise and had suggested that I should contact him to discuss further. I wanted to pick up the phone and call him right then, but I did not have his number and his signature was illegible. So, I would have to first contact the editor of the journal to get his number to pursue this issue.

Meanwhile, I was editing the book, *Pharmacophore Perception, Development, and Use in Drug Design,* and realized that these two papers would fit nicely into it. So, I contacted the editor of the journal, but instead of requesting the contact information of the reviewer, I told him that I was retracting the papers from his journal to be published elsewhere.

The idea of putting together the pharmacophore book came from a symposium that I had organized at one of the National ACS meetings concerning recent developments in pharmacophore modeling. A publisher contacted me a few weeks after the meeting and asked if I could get the speakers in my symposium to contribute to a book that I would edit. Concerned about the level of commitment, I had been categorically denying such requests over the years, but he was persistent. At one point, he told me that he had researched thoroughly and not a single book in the literature had the word "pharmacophore" in its title. This would be the first. He persuaded me, and I used this argument to persuade others to contribute to the first book on pharmacophores.[18] It was indeed a lot of work but it was fulfilling. Finally, the book published in 2000 with twenty-seven chapters, five of which included contributions from me, and two of which were the original GH-Score papers.[19,20]

One of the book's contributors was a well-respected scientist, Dr. Peter Willett, of the University of Sheffield in the UK. He was working on a project that involved evaluating various metrics to analyze similarity searches, and he decided to include the GH-Score in the study. He published a paper on that work in 2002.[21] The GH-score and one other metric called "cumulative recall" were among the top performing of those he evaluated. This gave the GH-Score some credibility, and people started asking about it. In his publication, Willett referred to the GH-Score as the "Güner-Henry Score". And the name stuck. How lucky can one get? The inventors of the GH-Score happened to have the initials G and H. The attribution changed from the "GH-Score developed by Güner and Henry," to the "Güner-Henry Score." Here I was, the kid who barely got a C in first-year calculus and had hated advanced math thirty years prior, now with his name associated with a mathematical formula.

Some years later, at one of the ACS national meetings, the Güner-Henry Score was prominently featured in about a dozen or so papers. My collaborator, Dr. Doug Henry, was a speaker in one of the symposia, and the conference chair introduced him as "the mysterious H of the GH-Score." During a reception at that conference, the chief-editor of the *Journal of Chemical Information and Computer Science* approached me to apologize. He explained that he had not assigned proper referees to the original two GH-Score papers that I had sent to his journal some ten years back. He asked me to please consider sending future papers to his journal.

* * *

I had Kurt join me on one of my backgammon trips to Detroit when he was fifteen. Whenever we went out for dinner as a group, Kurt would amaze the people around us with his knowledge of sports, stats, and gossip. At one point, while we were driving to a restaurant for dinner, one of the prominent players in the US backgammon scene, hearing Kurt spout his knowledge, turned around and asked Kurt just how old he was.

Kurt was into sports in general, but specifically basketball. He eventually picked Gonzaga University, I think primarily because of their basketball program, and also because of a modest merit scholarship they awarded him. Even though he was not playing basketball anymore, he still wanted to be close to the game. He got his BS and MS at Gonzaga while working part-time at various jobs, one of which involved being on the basketball floor, supplying stats to the press during the home games. For some years after he left Gonzaga, he still wrote articles and analyses in his blog after each game.

On one of my business trips to the UK I had Sibel, then fourteen, join me. It was a routine trip to Cambridge for meetings with my team and the software developers. A typical itinerary would be to leave California Monday morning to arrive at Gatwick Airport early Tuesday morning where a car would be waiting to take me to Cambridge. I would lower the seat-back and take a short nap during the three-hour drive to Cambridge, then check in to a hotel, shower, and head for the office. I would work in the Cambridge office for the rest of the week. Friday night, after work, I would take the train to London, check in to a hotel there, and have dinner at one of my favorite Turkish restaurants, the Sofra Restaurant in Mayfair. The waiters would recognize me and comment that it had been a while since my last visit. They probably thought I was a local.

Saturday morning, I always went to the half-price ticket booth at Leicester square to buy a ticket to one of the musicals. I would pick two plays while waiting in the line and buy tickets to the one with the best seats. As a single, I would usually find an excellent spot, like front center. Sunday morning, I would then return to San Diego. By staying over the Saturday night, I would get a big discount on the airline ticket and end up saving money in my travel account despite the extra day of accommodation in London.

With Sibel joining me, she quickly developed her own routine. She would spend time around the hotel while I was at work. After I returned from work, we would walk around Cambridge, then have dinner. During one of these walks Sibel asked me, "How come you are *still* married to Mom?"

It had been eleven years since Zeynep and I had first tried to divorce, when Sibel was three and Kurt was six and just starting school. After we decided to stay together for the kids, I felt that our marriage was merely a formality. Sibel must have clearly noticed our marriage's dysfunctionality, prompting her question on this trip. Hearing this, I wondered if we stayed together longer than we should have.

* * *

The University of California in San Diego had an extension program, the Executive Program for Scientists and Engineers (EPSE). It was designed for scientists and engineers who had no management experience but had reached a point in their careers where they became managers (or potential managers). It was like a mini-MBA for busy executives; a nine-month program that required a full-day attendance every Monday and occasional weekend days as well. Accelrys sponsored me and Dr. Marvin Waldman, my counterpart on the development team, to take this course. They not only paid for the tuition, but also allowed us to take Mondays off to attend the course for the following nine months.

Whereas I was responsible for product management and marketing for the cheminformatics and chemistry products, Marvin was responsible for the development of chemistry products. As such, Marvin and I ended up working closely together for the duration of my tenure at Accelrys. He is a bright and analytically gifted individual. We would almost always go head-to-head regarding which features to include in the next software release, trying to balance the cost versus benefits of each. Accelrys was now investing in us, perhaps to prepare us for some future executive roles in the company. I felt good about it. Those were the good old days.

The EPSE was beneficial to me. It covered topics from marketing and sales to pricing and packaging, leadership vs. management, team building, managerial economics, business management, and human resources, among others. I was able to use some of the concepts I learned right away to address challenges at work. For example, I organized a creative brainstorming meeting to figure out the future direction of our small-molecule modeling environment (called *Cerius-2*). Using several techniques that I learned from classes at EPSE, we had a productive meeting naming the priorities for the future of this system.

One of the more engaging part of the EPSE was taking part in a simulated business management competition called Capstone. A lot of fun, yes, but it also taught us about team building and management. This was like flight simulators that the pilots and astronauts use to gain experience dealing with different challenges and to develop good instincts. Here, we were to go through a simulated business management exercise. Each team would "take over" a struggling $100 million company and manage it for eight simulated years. The team would divvy up the roles of chief executive officer (CEO), finance, research and development (R&D,) and marketing/sales. Each member of the team had to make several critical decisions in their respective areas for every round (i.e., each simulated year). R&D had to prioritize product development resources, introduce new products, and adjust the existing products to make them more appealing to the market. Marketing decisions included which market segments to focus on, pricing, and how much of each product to produce. Then there were the financial decisions: where to invest, hiring and firing, whether to give dividends or take loans. The CEO would oversee each of the department's decisions to make sure that they aligned with the overall business strategy.

Our team did poorly. I was frustrated. We had agreed on a general strategy. We had set up the process to propose our decisions for our departments and how the decisions would be submitted. When I was on a business trip and could not attend the class, I sent my assigned decisions via email as we agreed. When I came back, I noticed that my recommendations had been changed contrary to what we had decided. According to the Tuckman model of *Forming, Storming, Norming, Performing* that we had learned about, we failed since our team did not abide by the *Norming*, because, apparently, we had not run through the *Storming* phase completely. I had elevated expectations because we did have a good strategy. But we could not implement the strategy since some members of the team were not on board, though they had initially accepted it.

This experience, though frustrating, was educational for me in understanding group psychology and how to deal with different people with different ambitions, skills, expectations, and needs. How to step in as a leader when needed. How we all needed to work with each other and the inevitable failure when a team was dysfunctional.

A while later, the instructor announced an international Capstone competition that was open to us since we had completed the course. I wanted to compete; I wanted to go all the way with a good strategy and a functional team. I approached Marvin, and we signed up. The first part of the competition involved each team competing against five computer teams with different business priorities. Capstone developed these virtual computer players, each with a slightly different business strategy, for training purposes. They used them for the international competition as well, perhaps since the virtual players provide an equal challenge for all the competitors. Each human team would compete against the same five virtual computer players.

The human teams submitted the business orders for each simulated year once per day. At the end of the day, the system released the annual report for each company and the decisions for the next simulated year to be considered. This went on for eight simulated years, and eight real days. At the end of the first part of the competition, after the eight days, the teams were ranked based on cumulative profits and the final stock price of the company. The top six teams became finalists. The finals took place on one Saturday, with each simulated year—with its various challenges and orders—compressed into an hour. In the finals, the six finalists competed against each other, not against virtual players. After eight hours, Capstone announced the champion team, again, based on cumulative profits and stock price.

One-hundred and forty-six teams competed from forty countries. Marvin and I felt we had an excellent strategy, if brutal and extremely hard to implement in real life. It involved selling off all the plants that were generating more than the optimum production we needed for the first year, laying off people working at those plants, then having the remaining employees work overtime at fifty-percent higher salary. We would use all the money gained from the sale of the plants and the lay-offs, and all the cash generated by the maximum amount of loans we could obtain, to invest in R&D to introduce three new products in the first year (rules limited us to maximum of three new product introductions over all eight rounds). By introducing all three in the first round, we benefited from their revenue for all subsequent rounds. We would have the advantage of having three more products than most of the competitors for at least the first few years. Once the new products were released, and as the business started growing again, we would hire back the people who lost their jobs in the first round. And, as the business continued to grow, we would continue to expand the workforce.

The strategy worked well. We were the highest scoring finalist. Among the six finalists, two of them were from the same university: Bilgi University in Istanbul, Turkey. We pondered whether they might cheat and work together in the finals, but soon rejected that idea. The timeline was so tight that they would barely have enough time to get their orders together, let alone figure out how to effectively collaborate. During the finals, every decision had to be made within an hour.

Considering his analytical strength, we would have Marvin make the most difficult and critical decisions. He was to spend forty-five minutes of the hour calculating the level of production for each product. He had developed algorithms to help determine this by analyzing what the market could bear, what the competitors were likely to do, what price level would be the most profitable, and the annual reports of all the competitor companies. I would oversee everything else: finance, sales, marketing, and R&D. In the last fifteen minutes of the hour, we would work together to enter the decisions for each department, then review the complete set of decisions, agree on them, and submit them.

At the end of the hour, the computer would use each company's decisions to assign the sales, profits, etc. and then print out each company's annual report. We would go through this process for eight straight hours. Marvin complained that he did not work this hard at his regular paying job.

At the start of the finals, our first-year orders were already decided since we had agreed upon our strategy, and we had all the information we needed to implement the orders. Once the first-year results were published, our stock price nosedived to an exceptional low, near zero, while everyone else was doing fine. The system did not like the fact that we took on a lot of high-interest loans, shut down plants, and laid off people. The stock price climbed back up to normal levels at the end of the second year when we had three added products with which we started to lead in the market. As we progressed with our strategy, the stock price continued to increase above everyone else's, and we took a solid lead.

Past mid-point, one of the competitors was consistently undercutting our sales in one segment by setting low prices. This was annoying. We needed to keep the prices at a profitable level, and this competitor was pricing as if they did not care about profits. So, we decided to deal with that competitor. Two rounds from the end of the competition, we priced the products in the low-end market at the minimum accepted value and flooded the market. Those products would not make a profit for us, but all the other competitors, unable to sell the same product at a higher price, would end up entering the last year with a huge inventory to deal with. It worked. Entering the last round of the competition, everyone but us was struggling. We had aggressively paid off our debts during the earlier rounds and were debt free with about $250 million cash in the bank. No one else had so much cash. Since only cumulative profits and stock price contribute to the final score and not the cash in the bank, we decided to give it all up as dividends. When the results were announced, our stock-price jumped from $15 per share to over $90, due to the generous dividends. We won, and by a large margin.

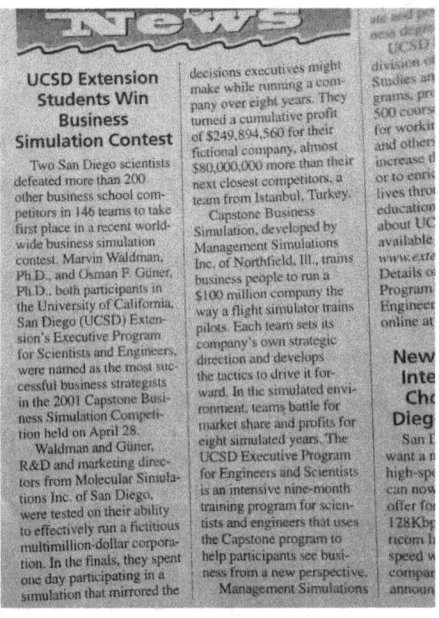

**NEWS**

**UCSD Extension Students Win Business Simulation Contest**

Two San Diego scientists defeated more than 200 other business school competitors in 146 teams to take first place in a recent worldwide business simulation contest. Marvin Waldman, Ph.D., and Osman F. Güner, Ph.D., both participants in the University of California, San Diego (UCSD) Extension's Executive Program for Scientists and Engineers, were named as the most successful business strategists in the 2001 Capstone Business Simulation Competition held on April 28.

Waldman and Güner, R&D and marketing directors from Molecular Simulations Inc. of San Diego, were tested on their ability to effectively run a fictitious multimillion-dollar corporation. In the finals, they spent one day participating in a simulation that mirrored the decisions executives might make while running a company over eight years. They turned a cumulative profit of $249,894,560 for their fictional company, almost $80,000,000 more than their next closest competitors, a team from Istanbul, Turkey.

Capstone Business Simulation, developed by Management Simulations Inc. of Northfield, Ill., trains business people to run a $100 million company the way a flight simulator trains pilots. Each team sets its company's own strategic direction and develops the tactics to drive it forward. In the simulated environment, teams battle for market share and profits for eight simulated years. The UCSD Executive Program for Engineers and Scientists is an intensive nine-month training program for scientists and engineers that uses the Capstone program to help participants see business from a new perspective.

Management Simulations

**News printed in the ComputerEdge weekly magazine, June 15, 2001**

Another immediate benefit of the EPSE course was that I could use the material from the course to construct a workshop for the product managers and product specialists in my group. Except for two members of my team who had MBAs, all the rest were PhDs. They were excellent scientists, but most of them did not have much business sense except for the bits they had learned on the job, just like me before the EPSE course. This workshop was perfect for them to get the basics of business concepts that they needed for their various jobs. The workshop was so successful that I decided to run it every year. It evolved into a three-day workshop where product managers from different departments would also attend. Eventually, I organized a five-day workshop that included a Capstone training and competition with the company's mid-level managers from all around the world attending.

\* \* \*

Towards the end of my tenure at Accelrys, I think I might have had my mid-life crisis. It took the form of a red Mustang convertible with black leather seats, one of the few indulgences in my life. I was shopping for a new car in 2005 but had never bought a new car before. I had always bought a used car, usually four or five years old. However, when I saw the bright red Mustang in the lot, I had to test drive it. I took the top down and drove it around the lot for a couple of blocks, and that was it. I was sold. The 2004 model was only a year old with twelve thousand miles on it, so new by my standards. This was at a time when my job at Accelrys was incredibly stressful, and I needed a distraction, something positive in my life.

Clearly my time with Accelrys provided many good memories. In nearly a decade there, I had grown, developing a deeper understanding of business management, and as a scientist. I made good money, traveled the world, became an American citizen, and bought a house (that I didn't quite feel I owned) and a Mustang convertible (that I truly enjoyed driving). I witnessed and shared the development, growth, and graduation of my children. In short, I had a wonderful time and memorable life experiences.

However, the reality was that I was eventually let go in a not-so-dignified manner, and then I had to figure out what to do next. I had always wanted to discover/design new drugs and a future job could help me accomplish this. Having been involved with the development of tools to help scientists design new drugs for sixteen years, I wanted to now use these tools and harness that experience to design drugs myself.

An idea I had for some time was to start my own consulting business providing contract research services. Why not?

# CHAPTER 8

# After 50: At Turquoise Consulting

## *San Diego, California, 2006-2010*

Once I left Accelrys, I was so intent on starting my sole proprietorship that I didn't spend much time searching for another corporate job. I went on just one interview with Tripos Inc. (a smaller competitor of Accelrys) for a vice president of Marketing position, and they ended up picking the other candidate. When I found out who that other candidate was, I completely agreed with them; it was a good pick. Meanwhile I focused on developing a business plan and a business model for my sole proprietorship, which I called Turquoise Consulting. I registered the name, posting an ad in a local newspaper. I got the rights for the "turquoisecons" domain name and set up a corporate bank account. I used Yahoo's small business package to develop my website. This was a lot of work, but I was enjoying it.

\* \* \*

Our two-story house in San Diego encompassed around 2,600 square feet. The second floor included a large master bedroom that had a hallway to a walk-in closet across from the "his-and-hers" faucets, a make-up area for "her," a large bathtub, full separate toilet, and a separate shower unit. Between the master bedroom and the children's rooms was the main bathroom. The children's bedrooms overlooked the front of the house, above the three-car garage, whereas the master bedroom looked out on the back yard. This quarter acre haven included an in-ground jacuzzi, sitting, dining, and barbeque areas, half a dozen trees, a large hammock, and a slight uphill incline with several eucalyptus trees. The entire back yard was tightly fenced to allow our Goldie to live outside with her "igloo" (a doghouse resembling an igloo) for shelter. The space was large enough to build a pool, a consideration when we bought the house. Concerned about maintenance and liability, I was able to persuade Zeynep not to build the pool. Back inside, downstairs had a large living area, dining area, guest area, a bar, a half-bathroom, and the laundry room.

When we had first moved in, a jar of apricot marmalade greeted us on the kitchen counter with a note from the previous owner telling us that it was from our apricot tree. From this prolific tree, we would collect lots of apricots during June and July. One year, we couldn't pick the apricots because we were in Turkey on vacation. When we came back, the apricots on the tree were large and plump, incredibly sweet, and delicious. We had been picking them too early all that time.

Once we got a call from some state organization asking permission to place a trap for the Mediterranean fruit fly on the strawberry guava tree in the front yard. Strawberry what tree? I hadn't even realized we had one. Apparently, that little messy sapling that produced a lot of odd fruit and messed up the front yard was an edible-fruit tree. And the strawberry guavas, we found out, were delicious. For years, we had missed out eating the delicious exotic fruits, again because of our ignorance.

It was a beautiful house, and we enjoyed it for many years. I commissioned as my home office another smaller room upstairs, between the master bedroom and the children's rooms.

\* \* \*

What logo would I use for my business? I downloaded a thirty-day evaluation copy of *WebLab Viewer* (PC-based software to draw chemical structures and create three-dimensional -renderings of them) and I created modeled images of common chemicals that have some significance in the biology and medical fields. I spent about month figuring out which structure to use in my logo and, in the end, picked the caffeine molecule. This chemical is obviously significant to humans. Half of us can't start our day without our morning caffeinated drink of choice, from coffee or tea to cola, and the other half of us drive the "caffeine-free" industry. With caffeine in my logo, I dispersed models of other important chemicals around my website, so each page had an image of at least one modeled molecule of interest as part of its design.

For the dot in the "i" of turquoise, I placed an evil eye, commonly displayed in Turkey to protect individuals, buildings, and businesses from the malevolent glare of anyone cursing you or wishing you bad luck. Most tourists who visit Turkey end up buying an evil eye as a souvenir. I'm not superstitious, but I was having fun and doing whatever I wanted in my own business, and why not play up my Turkish heritage? The turquoise color prominent in the graphic design is also of Turkish origin, and stares brightly from the traditional evil eye. One can find this color in sandy patches along the rocky Mediterranean coasts of Turkey. I also used a font with a decidedly Middle Eastern feel. A bit of chemistry, a touch of my cultural origin, and I had my logo.

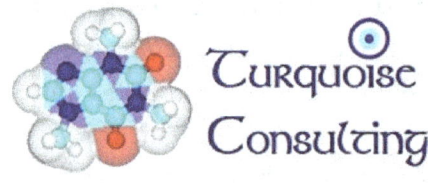

The logo of my new business, Turquoise Consulting

I also needed custom legal templates. For this, I reached out to my friend Lisa Balbes. She'd long had her own consulting business in St. Louis. She was helpful and generous. Using her suggestions, I gathered several documents for my own business templates and put them on my company letterhead, including for mutual non-disclosure agreements, invoices, and standard terms and conditions. With my website and business documents in place, my business was ready to start. I chose my fiftieth birthday, February 25, 2006, as my sole proprietorship's start date. A fresh start for my life after 50.

Up to this point in my working life, I'd never had a break between jobs. Starting with my doctorate in Virginia through my postdoc in Alabama to my jobs at Molecular Design Limited and Accelrys in

California, all the transitions included no breaks or interruptions, not a single day. So from my first job up to age 50, I had never been unemployed, with my next job already set up before the earlier one ended. Leaving Accelerys left me unemployed for the first time ever. With the start of my consulting business, I was starting an entirely new life chapter.

\* \* \*

The last couple of years at Accelrys was busy. Always rushing to meetings, completing tasks, nurturing projects, busy, busy, busy. Twice a week, I had a conference call at 7:00 a.m. with my team in the UK. It would be 3 p.m. over there so we would have several hours of overlap to work on issues.

Now, not quite yet having figured out how to manage my time, I had a lot of free time. I was both excited to explore new opportunities and scared about needing to pay the bills. I had a lot to figure out. I rolled up my sleeves and got to work on my new business, my new life.

With Turquoise Consulting, I intended to perform contract research and/or consulting for pharmaceutical or biotech companies using my fifteen plus years of experience in computer-aided drug design. In my corporate years, I had focused on developing methods to apply software tools that others used to design drugs. Now *I* wanted to use these tools to design drugs.

A few weeks after I started my business, Dr. Christian Lemmen, chief executive officer (CEO) of a German company, BioSolveIT GmtH, contacted me. Co-founded in 2001 by Dr. Lemmen, BioSolveIT provided software solutions and tools for drug design. He was expanding the business into the US market and was looking for someone to head up this effort. Would I be interested? It would be a bit of an effort to get the US Company incorporated, but once up and running, it could be a solid business.

When I asked about the candidate requirements, he said, "I am looking for an initiative-taking, self-motivated individual with business management experience, but also a hands-on scientist who knows enough about computers to maintain them and knows enough science to be able to demonstrate the company's products to American clients. At first, this branch will start as a single-person company, so I want someone with broad experience to tackle different aspects of the business."

This looked exceptionally good for me, the job requirements almost a carbon copy of my skillset. Just having started my own consulting business, and with all the work I had put in to get things up and running, and with all my built-up enthusiasm, I couldn't just give up on Turquoise Consulting so soon. I also really wanted to try the discovery and design of new drugs more than managing and supporting another software business. It was a dilemma. I wanted this job, a natural continuation of my career, yet I also wanted to give my consulting business a shot.

So I suggested a compromise that would be a partial win for both of us. I offered to find and recruit the person to manage their US branch for them. "Executive recruitment" ended up being the first formal project of Turquoise Consulting. I prepared all the paperwork. I received a third of the fee upfront as a retainer, another third upon completion of the interviews of the top three candidates, and the last third when the top candidate accepted the position and came onboard. Within several months I completed the project. BioSolveIT had their new US General Manager and Turquoise Consulting received three payments for the effort. This was not a drug discovery project that I was originally shooting for, but it was work nevertheless, and work that paid the bills.

In retrospect, I wondered if I might have made a strategic error in declining the job offer. It *was* perfect for me. I would have been able to use both my business management experience and my scientific background, as well as computer expertise.

But in the end, I don't think turning down the job was a mistake. I really didn't want to continue working for CADD software companies; I wanted to design drugs. And I would have a shot at that with my consulting business, now already off to a profitable start.

After I left Accelrys, the first thing I did when I got home was take off my wristwatch and my socks and settle into a relaxed mood in casual clothes. At work, I had always been in a hurry, always trying to make it to my overscheduled meetings, always racing around in my car to get where I was going. Once ousted from the corporate world, I decided that I would never rush anyplace again. I would leave early, give myself plenty of time, and if I ended up too early, I would stop by a coffee house and have some herbal tea or something to pass the time and relax. Having a convertible in San Diego (where the weather is always moderate) made my drives special. Now that I wasn't in a rush, I could fully enjoy driving the Mustang. If somebody wanted to cut in front of me, I would think, "Go ahead, by all means, I'm in no hurry." With this attitude, driving became a pleasure.

A company offered me a six-week consulting job doing market research. When I told the CEO that I no longer wore a watch or socks, he looked under the table and saw my flip flops under my slacks. It was fine with him. "As long as you aren't going into the labs," he told me, "I'm okay with you wearing your flip flops at work." Eventually, I started wearing socks again, but haven't worn a wristwatch since.

In a typical day in my life during this period, I would wake up early, take a shower, dress casually, and eat a light breakfast. Then I would spend the rest of the morning working on my projects. Sometimes I had to work on-site at a local company. Most of the time, I worked from my home office. At around noon, I would take my two-hour lunch break and jump into my convertible to drive to one of my happy places. There, I would set up my beach chair and enjoy a small lunch of a sandwich or a protein bar with a club soda or water and enjoy the scenery while reading a book. Some of my happy places—there were about a dozen of them—were a cliff in Del Mar, some of the great beaches in San Diego, somewhere high up in the hills with gorgeous ocean views. This was how I recharged my emotional batteries every day. I would then return home to do household chores, walk the dog, and perhaps take a short afternoon work. If Sibel was home after school, I would hang out with her. Usually though, Sibel would be working her afternoon shift at The Coffee Bean and Tea Leaf, and Kurt was away at college, so I had minimal time with the kids.

When I was working at Accelrys, or when I was traveling for business, I saw little of Zeynep. Once I started to work from home, our daily contact increased and so did the friction and stress of our relationship. There was no question that it was time for us to start working on our divorce. Since we agreed, we decided to go with divorce arbitration to keep ourselves out of the courts.

We found an arbiter and got the process started. The arbiter asked about payment for her services and explained that she would normally split the bill in two and send it to each of us monthly. Right there I made my first mistake: I told her I would pay the bills. Zeynep was not working at that time and was collecting an allowance for kitchen expenses from me anyway. But, soon after, she got a job and started earning her own money. Even then I was still paying all the bills and covering expenses. The arbiter was competent and efficient; she collected needed information and started to put together a settlement agreement.

Meanwhile, Zeynep and I decided to sell the house and split the proceeds. It had been about ten years since we bought the house, and we had a lot of equity accumulated to give each of us easily a five-or six-year period of relatively comfortable living. However, there was a tight window of opportunity. The market would be at its peak around May-June, when all the corporate executives coming to San Diego for new jobs would seek a house in a neighborhood with good schools.

The real estate agent we hired worked hard to get the house on the market before this window closed and was frustrated as Zeynep kept delaying the process for one reason or another. By the time we finally were able to put the house up for sale, the big buyers had already acquired their homes and demand had cooled. We received an off-season low-ball offer for the house, and at that point Zeynep decided she didn't want to sell it.

Meanwhile, also frustrated, our arbiter decided to quit. She said she couldn't move forward because Zeynep wouldn't respond to her questions and wouldn't meet with her. This was a setback, but we had a settlement agreement in good shape, and I figured we should be able to finish the process at the San Diego Divorce court with all the forms filled out. When we went to court, however, I discovered that while all my forms were complete, Zeynep's documents were not. I was frustrated and at my tipping point, so I insisted on getting a court date. If Zeynep wouldn't submit her documents by that date, we were to settle all this in court, and spend much of our savings on attorneys.

During the time we were working on our divorce, I decided to engage my kids in the process, mostly Sibel who was still at home but also Kurt too when he was in town. They would help me find an apartment. That way, when the day of our separation came, the kids wouldn't be surprised. Kurt was out of state at college, but Sibel had another year in high school. I explained to her that I would decide between two separate neighborhoods depending on whether she would live with me, as one was close to her high school. Otherwise, I would pick a place near downtown San Diego. The kids amused themselves—and me—by running internet searches and giving me links to potential apartments. I was proud of them.

I got a call from Zeynep's lawyer, an unexpected (to me) addition to the process. He aggressively tried to bully me with prepared statements about the value of the house and what needed to be done until I interrupted him. I told him that the number he was quoting was not the value of the house, but a low-ball offer we had received and that the actual market value of the house was significantly higher. That gave him pause. The incorrect low value was in Zeynep's interest since she wanted to buy me out. Once he realized I knew that he was a bit more civil when he started talking again. He would come up with an offer and call me back.

When he called me again about a month later, he sounded exasperated. He said Zeynep was demanding such-and-such and that I should pay such-and-such, etc. I said I would be happy to work with him on those issues, but after agreeing to his terms, within another few weeks, I suspected that he would call again with additional demands. I told him that I wouldn't deal with ever increasing demands. He said there would be no further demands and that Zeynep would sign the settlement agreement once her current demands were met.

We signed the settlement agreement a day before the court date. Zeynep bought my equity in the house. Sibel would stay with Zeynep, and I would pay child support until her eighteenth birthday. And we were done.

One silver-lining to this divorce settlement was that it eased my conscience. Zeynep's consistent handicapping of the process freed me from feeling guilty about the divorce. And with the outcome, I needn't worry if she would be okay. She had a job and a favorable settlement.

* * *

Sibel was exceptionally talented. Despite having earned a perfect score on the math SAT, she insisted on attending a liberal arts college. She was quadrilingual and a self-taught artist. She wanted to head East for college despite our efforts to dissuade her and keep her in California, where we could pay relatively affordable in-state tuition. She picked Boston College.

Sibel and I made the trip together to Boston College's beautiful campus. It was a Jesuit college (just like Kurt's Gonzaga), with a clean city campus. Because it sat on hills, the many steps to climb around campus would provide good exercise, and the cafeteria offered healthy food selections. I thought Sibel would enjoy her studies there. We found her dorm room, where her two roommates were already moving in with their parents' help.

We left to shop for necessities (sheets, pillows, clothes, pens, pencils, papers, calculator, personal items) and then returned to the dorm. Her roommates had already settled in, and we got Sibel settled in quickly too. After hanging out for another day and finding good dining options around campus, I returned to San Diego, leaving my little girl behind. In Skype meetings with her later, she complained about how cold it was. She said she had run out of layers to wear, and it was only October! Born and raised in California, she wasn't ready for winter. She eventually got good winter wear and stopped complaining about the cold.

Towards the end of her first year, Sibel decided she wasn't happy at Boston College. When I asked why, she said, "It's too white, too privileged, too preppy, and I really don't like the type of people on campus." She also didn't get along with her roommates. She got into Connecticut College for her sophomore year and asked, "Could you come and help me move and settle in at Connecticut College?" My little girl still needed me.

Connecticut College was more diverse for certain, with many students of color and international students as well. The campus was surrounded by natural beauty in the form of a 700-acre arboretum (as opposed to the marble temple-like setting of Boston College). It boasted nature trails, a forest, a lake. Its beautiful campus blended almost perfectly into its natural surroundings. Sibel scored a single room in the dorm (as did most students there). So she didn't have to worry about roommate problems like she had in Boston.

When I noticed a Walmart close to the campus, I was pleased that we could get all she needed in one stop. Boy, was I wrong! Sibel said she'd been boycotting Walmart because it wasn't paying its employees well. So, we spent a whole day running from store to store to find all she needed. As she settled in, she seemed to feel much better about the friendliness of the people here and the natural setting of the campus.

During her junior year at Connecticut College, taking advantage of a student exchange program, she studied abroad for a semester in Perugia, Italy. Then she did a summer internship at UNESCO's World Water Assessment Programme, which kept her in Italy for more than eight months altogether and left her fluent in Italian. She captured her experiences in Italy by sketching her surroundings in her sketch book every day. During the annual Umbria Jazz festival, she sat on a bench and sketched musicians. She was so focused on her pursuit that she didn't realize that passing tourists had formed a semicircle behind her and were watching her work. Without realizing it, she had become part of the festivities.

\* \* \*

I was living alone in an apartment in San Diego after my divorce was finalized. One day when I was taking a shower, I noticed a big spider, skinny with long legs, in the bathtub. I tried to shoo it away by splashing water on it, but it managed to move away and stay dry. I decided to ignore it and went on with my shower. When I was drying up, I noticed that it was still there. I decided that since it managed to survive so far, it deserved to live; and that started our long coexistence. I called it "George."

Sometime later, Sibel, spent the weekend with me. I heard a shriek from the bathroom. I rushed there, half expecting that she had fallen and broken a bone or something. She was pointing towards the bathtub at the big spider. I was relieved that she was okay and introduced her to George. I said, "You should just ignore him and take your shower; George knows how to avoid splashes." George the spider lived happily in my apartment until my departure for my first relocation back to Turkey in 2010.

\* \* \*

It took three years for me to secure a contract research project with a pharmaceutical company, an exceedingly long time for a small business to go without the work for which it exists. Instead, I worked on short-term research projects, consultations, market research, and scientific presentations and workshops that supplied a small income, sometimes in the form of an honorarium. My vision of lucrative projects for contract research to pharmaceutical companies was a bit delusional. I came to realize my limitations. While I was enthusiastic about research, I hated spending time on the marketing and business development required to get new business. This is something many people with sole proprietorships deal with, I suppose.

Once I realized that I would not be able to generate a sustainable income through consulting alone, I found a way to generate supplementary income through my new hobby, bridge. I started learning how to play bridge as a teen in Turkey. Even though I enjoyed the game, it was never a serious affair, and my skills slowly faded over the years. This was the case until my fiftieth birthday. Once I started my own business,

I had a flexible schedule, and I remembered how I used to like bridge as a kid. I thought this might be a good time to relearn the game and perhaps take it more seriously. I searched for a bridge club nearby that also had classes. I signed up and started my bridge career.

My first shock was the sight of bidding boxes. I had never seen one before and was amazed by how easy they made the bidding process. The bidding systems themselves surprised me next. They were like a foreign language. I had learned a simple system called Goren when I was a teenager, but now no one was playing that system. Many players had not even heard of it.

I started taking some classes and playing at beginners' bridge games. Pretty soon I was getting good at it. One of my favorite partners at the beginners' games was Susan, an accountant. During the three months leading up to the April 15 tax-filing deadline, she couldn't play due to her crammed workdays. When she returned to the club a few months later and asked about me, our fellow beginners told her that I was now playing with the big boys and girls in the big room. While she was gone, I had exceeded the 50 masterpoint limit to play in the beginners' games. In bridge, as in chess, a player's scores in formal games contribute to a recorded, ongoing ranking, known as "rating" in chess and "masterpoints" in bridge. The more you win, the more masterpoints you accumulate. And they don't let the higher scoring hawks loose on the sparrows still learning the game by organizing games limited to players within a certain masterpoint range.

Soon after, I was regularly playing three to four times a week and consistently improving my game. As I improved, I started to partner with stronger players and garner occasional wins in club-level tournaments. I also started to get new partnership requests to travel to play in "regional" and "sectional" tournaments with these more serious upper-level players. There were also competitive team games. In short, bridge offered a bevy of exciting opportunities, and I was having fun.

Within six months of rededicating myself to the game, people started congratulating me in passing. I gracefully accepted their kudos, though I didn't know the reason for them. I assumed they were referring to my win the previous week. The praises continued for some time; obviously, something else was going on. Since I didn't ask at the beginning and pretended to know the reason for their tributes, it was too late to ask later. Eventually I figured out that it was for my standing in the North American Masterpoint races.

I had started playing the beginner bridge games in November 2005. By the time I finished the year two months later, I had 2.7 masterpoints. The American Contract Bridge League tracks individual's masterpoints and stratifies players at the start of each year:0 5 masterpoints for beginners, and upwards with ranges of 5-20, 20-50, 50-100, 100-200, etc. Since I started the year 2006 with 2.7 masterpoints, I classed as a Rookie. American Contract Bridge League posted the standings of all North American players in the Bridge Bulletin. I topped the Rookie category. I remained on the top of the list for 11 months and was surpassed by a Canadian player in the last month of the year, so finished second. Finishing the year as a runner up was good enough for me to start a "bridge résumé" that opened doors to various other opportunities. By the end of 2007, I was a club director and a bridge teacher. As a certified club director, I could run sanctioned bridge games and get a commission based on the number of players in the game. As an accredited teacher, I would be able to collect half of the revenues from students' fees (with the club getting the other half) for the classes I taught.

Once I was a certified director, I started to direct games at a large club in San Diego. As an accredited bridge teacher, I generated income from teaching bridge classes too. This activity supplied a much-appreciated supplemental income while my consulting business struggled. One year, my tax filings showed that I generated more income from bridge than from my consulting business. This says less about how well I was doing in bridge than about how poorly my consulting business was doing.

My bridge home base was Adventures in Bridge, a large San Diego club, listed year after year as one of the most active in the US. Some days, three separate games ran simultaneously in three different rooms: a beginner's game in the small room; an intermediate game (people below 299 masterpoints, or non-life-masters) in the medium room;

and an open game in the large room. I was directing Wednesday afternoon games and Friday morning games. The Friday game included a breakfast buffet, and it was crowded; we would have over twenty tables, on average, usually over 100 players, and typically two separate sections. Because I lived very close to the club, I would be on the call list to fill in if there were an odd number of players or pairs.

One evening I received a call from my boss at the bridge club. He asked if I could join him to fill a half table with an odd number of pairs in a game. Otherwise, one pair would end up sitting out each round. My boss always wanted to fill up half tables so that no one ended up sitting out. I was available and joined the game. I partnered with my boss to play against two charming ladies. They had a blast during the enjoyable game, with my boss, as the owner of the club, entertaining them throughout.

I noticed one of the ladies, Sevilla, gave me a sideways look. An excellent player, she was brunette, tall, and slim. The combination charmed me. Was there a possibility of romance in that glance? Recently divorced, I was a free agent. But I hadn't dated anybody for close to thirty years. How was it even done these days?

I harnessed the courage to ask her, and Sevilla and I started dating. We also enjoyed playing as partners. Because of her 2,500 Masterpoints (to my newbie 400) we could only play at open games. In one of the large games, to my amazement, we won. We faced strong players, some grandmasters with over 15,000 masterpoints in the game. I thought this win was a good omen. We were fond of each other, and our relationship evolved. At its peak, we were practically living together, splitting time between two locations. She would stay with me close to Adventures in Bridge several nights a week on days I was working at the club, and I would stay with her close to her club for several nights on days she was running her games. She owned a small bridge club in Encinitas, and I would help her run the games there.

Our bridge game was also going well, but we occasionally disagreed over a particular play. I didn't understand why she would dig in to defend a position rather than show flexibility. She was a strong player, and she could afford to take an occasional chance, but she would stick to her guns. This happened several times.

One day she showed me a spreadsheet that she had created, recording all her income and expenses, projected into the future. She had divorced several years earlier and was receiving alimony, coded in her spreadsheet along with her estimated income from bridge. She would run automatic calculations and could project "what if" scenarios. For example, she had purchased an industrial property on the East Coast that became a source of lease income from a medical instrument company. What would happen if she sold that business? How would the loss of the rental property income affect her finances? What would happen when the alimony checks ended? All these scenarios were in the spreadsheet. I was flabbergasted. In my view, no mere mortal could generate such a sophisticated spreadsheet.

Meanwhile, our arguments at the bridge table increased. After our relationship ran its course over six months and we decided to separate, I learned that she was dyslexic.

Now I got it! Her heavy reliance on bridge play rules *and* the spreadsheet! Yes, most people couldn't generate such a spreadsheet, but many a dyslexic person could. While people may associate dyslexia with learning disabilities and reading challenges, I think of Thomas Edison, Albert Einstein, Leonardo da Vinci—from the long list of dyslexic people with remarkable achievements. I have a tremendous respect for people with dyslexia.

I have developed an opinion that dyslexic people were dominant, and thus "normal" up to about six thousand years ago. With the invention of the alphabets and their evolution, our species took about two thousand years to learn how to read effectively, and society increasingly perceived people who could easily learn to read as normal. Our brains weren't wired to read, so we had to develop new neural connections and routes to learn the necessary skills. Since these connections weren't in the genes transferred to the next generations, each generation would have to learn reading from scratch. Dyslexic people favor their dominant right brain, which sees associations effectively but doesn't read easily.

We're now able to teach our children how to read in about five to six years from birth. While the ability to read doesn't transfer to following generations, genes associated with dyslexia can. Perhaps nature knows what it's doing. While, like everyone, each dyslexic person is unique, because of the dominant use of their right brain, people with dyslexia tend to be more creative, more resourceful, and able to recognize patterns more capably than non-dyslexic people. They can achieve great things, especially if given a school environment that is more nurturing than hostile.

In one of my bridge classes, I noticed I had a dyslexic student. She was having a hard time in evaluating the value of a hand. So after class, I developed a flowchart on how to evaluate a hand for her. Using this firmly structured process, she could go through it and correctly value a hand. If I gave some hands as a challenge to the class, most of the students would get the right answers about nine out of ten times and very quickly. My dyslexic student took more time evaluating the hand against the flow chart, but she got it right every time.

Meanwhile, I had exceeded the total number of masterpoints to become a Life Master in bridge, though I still needed 0.4 Gold masterpoints, which I could only earn in National and Regional tournaments. For four months I retained this status because I was not travelling to play in those big tournaments. Eventually, I relented and joined a woman, let's call her Mary, who also needed Gold masterpoints, and another a couple who were very strong bridge players. The four of us leased a condo in Las Vegas where we participated in a regional tournament. The condo was beautiful: fully furnished, large kitchen, three bedrooms, and a large jacuzzi. The first day of the tournament, we played in a knockout team game, and because we made it to the finals, we collected a little over 13 Gold masterpoints. So, both Mary and I became Life Masters on the first day of the tournament.

The next day, we played in a two-session (morning and afternoon) game in the open division. Because we had already earned the gold points we needed and the pressure was off, we were relaxed and having a great time. That's probably what gave us the courage to play in the open section (as opposed to in a limited section, below 500 masterpoints). In the open section, we would likely rank the lowest. In the morning session we placed in the middle of the pack. The team leading the game included one of the top players in the US, Mark Itabashi, in partnership with one of his students. Itabashi had over 35,000 masterpoints at that time. In the afternoon session we played against this formidable team in one of the later rounds, and, to our amazement, thanks to the mistakes the student made, we handed them two low boards (meaning we were the top pair amongst the players of those two boards). Our overall tournament finish was respectable and earned us some more Gold masterpoints, but the highlight of the day was knocking Itabashi out of first place.

We were elated, drunk with our accomplishment. When we went back to the condo, the other couple were out, probably playing an evening game. We tried the jacuzzi and, having no bathing suits, skinny dipped. That started my second recent attempt at a romantic relationship. We weren't very compatible, but the ecstasy of a successful performance at the tournament was a powerful aphrodisiac. This relationship lasted only six weeks.

There must be something about the number six with me. My first relationship as a divorcé lasted six months, the second six weeks, and the third one would last close to six years. All three were from the bridge club.

I detest first dates, where you each try to impress the other, superficially acting a role while trying to figure out the other person. Whereas in the bridge club, people would get to know each other naturally, observing each other over time and sometimes under pressure. No need for superficial first dates! So no surprise that my first relationships after the divorce were all with the people from the bridge club.

Vicki was a student in one of my beginners' classes. She was tall with short brown hair and a beautiful smile. She wore reading glasses with colorful rims and actively participated in class. She took the second, follow-up class as well. After the end of that course, I didn't see her again for a while.

One day when I went to the club for my scheduled game, I found a message from my partner that he wouldn't be able to play that day due to a last-minute engagement. As I looked around for the club director to see if anyone else needed a partner, Vicki walked into the room. I asked if she had a partner, and she didn't. I asked if she would like to play with me, and she did. We had a nice game, and she felt good about the experience. After the game she offered me a ride to my apartment (the club was walking distance from my apartment, so I didn't have my car). I asked if she wanted to come up for a drink and, to my surprise, she said okay. We enjoyed each other's company, and that was the beginning of an on-and-off six-year relationship.

\* \* \*

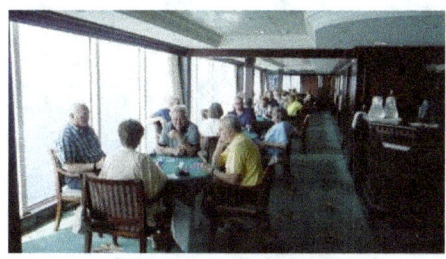

**Bridge games on a cruise ship**

In 2008, I started teaching bridge and running sanctioned games on cruise ships in exchange for food and accommodations—a free cruise for playing and teaching bridge and being a guest lecturer. I eventually stopped playing bridge in clubs but continued to teach on cruise ships, including one that circumnavigated the globe in one-hundred-eleven days in 2016, where, as I discuss in chapter 12, I gave seventy-one bridge lessons and ran about the same number of sanctioned games.

As a bridge director on a cruise ship, I could invite another guest. On one of the cruises, I had Sibel join me. This "Holy Lands" cruise started in Piraeus Greece before continuing to Santorini and Patmos Islands (Greece); Kuşadası (Turkey); Haifa and Ashdod (Israel); Alexandria and Port Said (Egypt); and then Sorrento and Rome (Italy). It was great to have Sibel with me. She was able to contribute to bridge play since I had earlier taught her how to play. When my wife and I were separated and going through our divorce proceedings, Sibel would spend every other weekend with me, and we also had Monday evenings to hang out. These Monday nights we would have dinner then go to the bridge club to play.

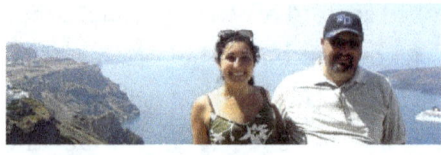

**With Sibel at Santorini, during the Holy Lands cruise**

Since she knew the basics of the game, she came to the rescue on the cruise when we ended up with an odd number of players and she could fill in at sanctioned afternoon games. She loved the cruise, the excursions, the fine dining, and the shows. Sibel was the co-captain of the speech-and-debate team at Torrey Pines High School when she was merely a junior. Articulate and generally knowledgeable, she would amaze our table mates over dinner with her sophisticated conversation, especially about environmental issues.

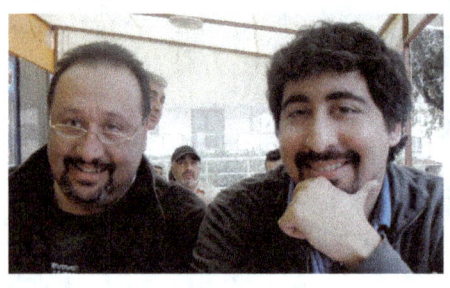

**With Kurt**

Kurt joined me on one of my bridge cruises too. By now, he was an adult working on his PhD in history at the University of Utah. He worked several jobs during his doctorate studies, mostly as adjunct faculty in the community colleges around Salt Lake City, where he developed a polished and professorial talking style. During the dinners on the cruise ship, he would mesmerize our tablemates with his deep understanding of politics and history.

With Sibel and Kurt on the cruise ships with me, I sat back and watched my kids gather respect and compliments from the people around us. Some of those compliments would trickle down to me. "You must have done something right to have raised such wonderful kids," people would say. The truth is their mother Zeynep had always focused more on their wellbeing. Despite our poor marriage, I had always appreciated her devotion to our children.

Everyone has a bucket list. High on mine for a long time was ballroom dancing, yet I kept avoiding it. I didn't think I would fit in. I was overweight and probably too clumsy as well. But my life after fifty involved trying things outside of my comfort zone. Eventually I signed up for a beginners' ballroom class in San Diego. It took me several classes to relax and start enjoying myself. At first, I didn't take part in the associated free dance parties since I knew only a few beginners' moves and still felt out of place. But over time, I felt more at ease with dancing. Vicki—a good dancer—and I attended some of the dance parties.

Vicki also joined me on a cruise, a short one called the "Mexican Riviera" cruise, a round trip from Los Angeles. We enjoyed the shore excursions to coastal towns of Mexico. One night on the ship, ballroom music played in the main atrium that had a small dance floor. Several couples were dancing. The atrium had three or four levels and people stood at the railings of the atrium enjoying the music and watching the people dancing. Vicki suggested we join the dancers and, just as we strolled out, cha-cha music started playing—one of our favorites. So, we danced to the familiar rhythms of the cha-cha and had a lot of fun. The next day, during lunch, some of the people at the table recognized us and told us that we were the best dancers on the floor the previous night. Which meant Vicki was excellent as people always watch the lady in ballroom dancing, the gentlemen's role being merely to show her off.

* * *

Monday nights I started playing in a Pro-Am game (for both professionals and amateurs) at the bridge club. Because Monday nights were my social time with Sibel, she would also come to the club and play at the beginners' game in the small room. She had developed a good partnership with another beginner player, and they ended up winning several of the games. In the Pro-Am game, each pair would consist of a mentor and a mentee. My mentor was Dr. Jeremy Fields. A biology professor at San Diego State University, he was tall, olive-skinned, bespectacled, and had about 3,000 masterpoints. I think he was from a Caribbean Island, but I don't remember which. On Monday nights he would critique my play and make suggestions. At the end of the game, we would go through each of the boards and figure out the best plays. I was learning a lot from Jeremy. We would also play occasional pick-up games, but Monday nights was when I would get rigorous training and coaching from him. Usually, Sibel would finish her game before ours, so she would sit with us and listen to Jeremy's analysis of the boards. The beginners' game used exactly the same boards, so the analyses benefited her as well.

One day I heard, Jeremy had a stroke while riding his bicycle along a nature trail. He sat next to his bicycle, but with few people around, by the time someone noticed something was wrong, crucial time passed, and his hospitalization and treatment were delayed. Jeremy lost his speech and the function of his right hand. When I learned about it, I was devastated. I visited him at his home and discovered, sadly, that despite his having speech therapy, we could communicate only with great effort. I would try to guess what he was trying to say, and he would approve or disapprove. It was a slow progress, but we were able to communicate a little in this manner.

A British couple in the medical field also shared the love of bridge with Jeremy, so the four of us would meet at least once every other week at his house to try some physical activities and some games. Because verbal communication wasn't possible, we played dominoes to assess his mental status. He beat us all. When we finally started playing bridge, it seemed like he was doing fine. Jeremy and I decided to go play the Pro-Am game the next Monday night. The British couple were going to England and would not be there.

I picked up Jeremy from his house, and we went to the club. Everybody was overjoyed to see him back. We played a good game and finished third. The British couple monitored the club web site until the results were posted and were happy to learn that we did so well.

* * *

It was my fifty-third birthday, and the weather was exceptionally good. So, I opened the front door to let the air in and was busy washing dishes when Kurt showed up. He was in town, and I had been expecting him to come over to hang out with me and Vicki for my birthday. A little later, Vicki came over and told me that they'd organized a surprise activity for my birthday. So, we got into her car, and she started driving. Neither of them would tell me what the surprise was.

We drove south towards the Mexican border. I guessed that a big outlet shopping center near the border was our destination. When we passed the last exit before Tijuana, I started panicking. I said "Where are we going? We can't enter Mexico. I don't have my passport with me." Then from the back seat Kurt produced our passports. Apparently, Vicki conspired with Kurt, who stole my passport. We had breakfast in Rosarita, lunch in Ensanada, and had a blast of a day excursion in Mexico, a wonderful and memorable birthday surprise. It was late at night when we returned home.

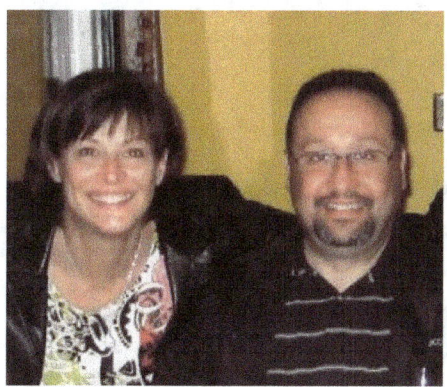

**With Vicki**

A few months later, when Vicki's birthday was approaching, I was determined to match her exceptional birthday gift. I organized an excursion to Coronado, a peninsula across the Bay from San Diego, famous for its golf courses, the Hotel Del Coronado, and beaches. We spent the afternoon at the beach across from the Hotel Del, where several movies had been filmed, including in 1959 *Some Like it Hot,* starring Marilyn Monroe, Jack Lemmon, and Tony Curtis. The fine and soft sand there makes it probably the best beach in the San Diego area, perfect for walking barefoot. Following beach fun, we had dinner in Coronado and made our way to my surprise main event, a Venetian-style sunset gondola ride with chocolate covered strawberries and a bottle of red wine. We had a wonderful time. Later, Vicki posted pictures on Facebook, saying it was the most romantic day of her life.

\* \* \*

Sometime in 2009, my consulting business had a breakthrough. Johnson & Johnson Pharmaceuticals offered me a contract-research position. Finally! This was exactly what I wanted to do with my business. Perhaps, Turquoise Consulting would be fine after all.

# CHAPTER 9

# At J&J Pharmaceuticals

*La Jolla, California, 2009*

Johnson & Johnson Pharmaceutical Research & Development, LLC (J&J), in La Jolla, California, contracted me for a three-month research job with its molecular modeling team. As a consultant I would help the team to find some new, biologically active chemical entities to overcome the safety concerns of the project's current active compounds. Besides my specialty in pharmacophore modeling, I had added skills to tackle exactly this kind of a problem. The main three-dimensional (3D)-searching software at J&J, however, was the latest new pharmacophore modeling software, *Phase* from Schrödinger, Inc. I was not familiar with this system. The main developer of *Phase* at Schrödinger was one of the original developers of Accelrys' *Catalyst*. The concept was similar, which would make my learning easier. My boss-to-be at J&J arranged for me to be trained on the software at the local Schrödinger office before my first day on the job. I gladly spent a week learning the software. Just as *Catalyst* was an upgrade from *MACCS-3D* when I moved from MDL to Accelrys, *Phase* was an upgrade from *Catalyst*. So, I learned the latest generation of the technology before I started my work at J&J.

\* \* \*

Monday mornings were my favorite days, not only because they provided a fresh start for the week, but also because my search results from big weekend jobs would have finished, and new results tend to bring new excitement to research. I was putting my *Phase* training to good use. J&J's corporate database was available in *Phase* format, but it was physically located in Philadelphia, about 2,700 miles and three time zones away. A pharmaceutical company's corporate database of proprietary molecules is one of their most valuable assets: the corporate treasures. I think they were hesitant to send a copy of the database to La Jolla. Considering it takes an average of about sixteen years and costs over a billion dollars to develop one new drug, chemical structures in corporate databases are protected like gold deposits in a Swiss bank. So, I had to access the database at its location in Philadelphia.

This geographical gap supplied our first challenge. To solve it, J&J set up an account for me with the computational chemistry group in Philadelphia, where I could direct my search jobs through a command line interface (the blank space on a screen where you type instructions in computer code). I would send my command file to Philadelphia through a secure connection and run the jobs over there. Once they completed, I would download the results to my workstation in La Jolla and analyze them in my local environment. This solution was convoluted but workable. I would send small search jobs before I left work at the end of each day. The next morning, I would download the results and continue with my work. This way, my computer use in Philadelphia was confined to evenings when everyone else was in their homes and it would not affect their work. Friday nights, however, I could send larger jobs that would run the entire weekend. This left me eager for Monday mornings when I would download the weekend results to my local workstation and enjoy whatever new insights they might contain.

These pharmacophore searches can take a long time and use abundant resources. The 3D structural searches align the compounds in the database to the pharmacophore model, considering multiple conformations for each compound. Once the software iterated all the conformations in the database, it would reevaluate close misses by flexibly aligning them (i.e., tweaking their rotatable bonds on the fly to see if a new conformation might exist that matched a model not stored in the database). Assessing those flexible large compounds simply took a long time. The more of these large flexible compounds in a given segment of the database being searched, the longer the process took, with the more memory required.

One Monday morning, I started down the stairs to the lab. I have always wondered why the molecular modeling lab sat underground. It felt to me like a Faraday's cage, which is an enclosure to block electromagnetic fields. Eventually I figured out why my cell phone's battery would always die before the end of the day. It was constantly searching for a satellite connection, sapping its energy. It could not find a satellite to connect to *because* we were underground. It was intentionally a Faraday's cage, probably to help keep their digital molecular wealth secure. After that, I made sure that my cell phone was turned off before entering the lab.

On this day, when I opened the door to the lab, things felt different. With palpable tension in the air, people stopped what they were doing and stared at me. I looked at my boss, and she pointed to her office.

What was going on? Were they considering firing me? It would take them more time to let me go than was left on my contract. Also, why would they do that? They were satisfied with my progress. So, bewildered, I went in my boss's office and sat on the chair she pointed at. She said she had several voice messages from the Philadelphia office asking about the jobs I was running on their main server.

One of the weekend jobs I ran had not finished by Monday morning. Some larger or more flexible compounds must have been in this batch, so it needed more resources than usual. My boss told me that the computer on which I was running my jobs was the main administrative computer everybody was connected to and used for day-to-day activities. My job likely started pulling resources from other areas in the computer, hogging both computer memory and disk space. By the time people arrived at work in Philadelphia, when they logged in to their accounts to check their email, the system was sluggish. I imagine that the information technology team (IT) was inundated with phone calls and messages from frustrated people trying to start their workday, and they were trying to figure out what was going on.

They soon realized a job by someone named Osman in the computational chemistry group had taken over most of the available resources in the computer that was fundamental to keeping their business running. I hope it did not take too long for someone in IT to remember that they had given an account to a consultant named Osman from the La Jolla group in California to access their local database. With the time zone difference, if they had called the La Jolla office, no one would have been there to pick up the phone. Luckily, by the time my boss arrived at her post in La Jolla, my job in Philadelphia had finally completed, and it gracefully released the resources it had taken over. Soon everything was back to normal in Philadelphia.

My boss said I was no longer allowed to use this main computer for my projects. I deserved this practical reprimand, a minor rap on the knuckles. Instead, she directed me to send my future jobs to another computer in Philadelphia reserved for research. I had not even realized I had a choice. I contacted the support desk at Schrödinger and learned how to identify that specific server so I could direct my jobs to it. I felt bad for inconveniencing my host.

I successfully completed my work at J&J. By the end of my term, I recommended that J&J asses for the specific biological activity close to a thousand compounds from its internal database. Later, I found out that nearly half of those compounds proved to be active, though most were already known to them since I was searching through their own corporate database. However, a few new active compounds from my list were ones that they had not expected to be active, which they could now pursue. These were excellent findings that boosted their research. My co-workers at J&J had been supportive, and I truly enjoyed my short time there.

The money I made from this contract conveniently paid all my outstanding bills and, as a bonus, left enough for me to take my two kids to Turkey for a month to visit our extended family. As usual, the kids loved the trip. The delicious Turkish food; meeting with their grandma, aunt, cousins, and interacting with them; swimming at the beach, playing backgammon, and taking long walks along the coastline: it was all a blast for them. Vicki also came to Marmaris for a week. It was her first trip to Turkey, and we had fun together. Life was good.

I found my experience at J&J valuable. I was finally able to directly participate in active drug research using the sophisticated machinery with which I was so familiar. I was finally able to practice what I had been preaching. I could use this successful experience to pitch other companies for further consulting opportunities, making this type of work my specialty. With a proven track record, I could adjust my business model to highlight this ability. Surely, now new doors would open. When I returned from Turkey, I found a message from my former boss at J&J requesting a call back. She said they had kept my work area as is, including the computer, workstation, passwords, and, if I would be interested, they would like to hire me again for another three months. This was exactly what I was looking for to stabilize my consulting business. I said I was okay with that, so they sent the contract request to headquarters in New Jersey. Since I was vetted already, they expected the contract to come through quickly.

But then I didn't hear back from them. I later learned that J&J leadership had made a strategic decision to move out of the area I happened to be working in. My timing sucked. Here I thought my business was about to move toward growth and prosperity, but I was back at the beginning. Time to move on.

\* \* \*

I had always considered returning to Turkey following my US retirement, which was then thirteen years off, but I started to think that I might not be able to survive in the US until then without a stable income. Alternatively, I could start to tap my retirement funds (a rollover IRA) in only six years. So, if only I could manage to support myself for another six years, I would then be able to pay myself a salary.

*Or*, I could move my consulting business to Turkey! This way, I'd be close to my extended family, and I could live comfortably thanks to

a lower cost of living there. My new business model could be to identify new drug leads for pharmaceutical and biotechnology companies
in Turkey.

I gave myself until January 1, 2010 to find more work in the US.
If I didn't get a new contract-research job by then, I would shut down
the business in San Diego and move to Turkey. The deadline passed
without a bite, and it took me three months to get my affairs in order.
I sold or donated to local charities my furniture, appliances, electronics,
kitchenware, and most of my clothing. The only things I shipped to
Turkey were about a dozen paintings, twenty-five boxes of books, and
some incidentals and personal items. After I vacated my apartment, I
stayed with Vicki for about a month until my flight. I gave my wristwatch to Kurt but kept my flip-flops. I bought a one-way ticket to
Ankara and left in April.

# CHAPTER 10

# At Turkuaz Danışmanlık

*Ankara, Turkey, 2010-2012*

The trip to Turkey was straightforward. After giving myself several days to settle in and acclimate to the time zone, ten hours ahead of California, I started to work. First order of business: getting the Turkish version of Turquoise Consulting ("Turkuaz Danışmanlık") up and running. An accountant friend helped me set up the company. The local bureaucracy dragged on for a few months, as opposed to only a few weeks in San Diego. I duplicated the web pages and translated them into Turkish, a lot of necessary work that made Turquoise Consulting webpages bilingual. My logo's evil-eye migrated to below the "s" in Danışmanlık.

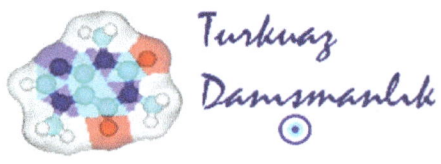

The logo of my consulting business in Turkey

Several friends in academia familiar with my past work enthusiastically received my "permanent" relocation to Turkey. Some invited me to speak at local conferences, giving me the opportunity to promote my emerging consulting business, which people seemed excited about. I chaired a session at a conference in Ankara, and I invited my ex-boss Scott Kahn, then chief information officer at Illumina Inc., to present the latest developments in the biomedical field. After the conference, I took him around Ankara, where he was particularly impressed with the Anatolian Civilizations Museum. It was good to catch up with Scott.

Scientists attending these meetings in Ankara told me they were glad to see I had moved my business to Turkey and that my skills were much needed to help bring a new focus to the pharmaceutical industry there. Unfortunately, most of the large companies in this sector in Turkey were subsidiaries of the larger multinational pharmaceutical companies. These parent companies had their research centers elsewhere, and they did not seem to want yet another research center in Turkey. Overall, more enthusiasm than genuine business opportunity existed, aggravated by my reluctance to spend time on business development and marketing. I did make some effort and met with industry executives and scientists. The younger scientists wanted to be involved in drug design and discovery, but nothing much came out of these meetings. The Turkish pharmaceutical sector didn't seem ready for someone like me in 2010. My timing and my prospects for success were poor.

* * *

Meanwhile, I applied for a new Turkish Identification Card, since the old one indicated that I was married. I filled out the form and specifically marked that I was divorced. When the new card arrived, it still showed me as married. According to Turkish law, Zeynep and I *were* still considered married despite the divorce being completed in the US. I had to hire an attorney to translate the US divorce documents and validate that the US divorce was compatible with Turkish law, and we would divorce again in Turkey. In the process, they would ship forms to Zeynep for her signatures. "What happens if Zeynep ignores the forms" I asked. They would send another set after three months. "What happens then?" They would send the material to the Turkish consulate in Los Angeles and have them verify everything. I left it to my lawyer to complete the process and a year later, our divorce was finalized in Turkey as well.

* * *

My consulting business received some support from Schrödinger in the form of a four-month free license to their small-molecule modeling system *Maestro*, including my new favorite, the *Phase* system. In exchange, I could be called upon to show the software to their prospects in Turkey. Since I could not afford the license fees for the software, I had only four months to do some interesting work. This kept me entirely busy during that time. I wanted to assess whether I could design compounds that would fit the active site of an enzyme, before and after a mutation modified the enzyme. The aim was to avoid drug-resistance caused by such mutations. Success would mean we could design drug resistance-resistant drugs. Such a solution could be critical when fighting a new virus, for example, which tends to mutate and evade existing treatments that worked with the earlier strains.

I sought to prove the concept with *Phase*. I evaluated a list of compounds that inhibit two different active sites on related enzymes. If these two different sites started as the same site with one of them altered through a mutation, then we might be able to develop a solution for drug resistance by identifying a compound active on both sites.

For the proof-of-concept, I developed a series of pharmacophore models that represent compounds known to bind to an enzyme site called phosphodiesterase (PDE) IV, and another series known to bind to PDE III. Then I merged some of the models to retrieve the compounds that fit into the active sites and align themselves with the complementary features of *both* receptors. Sure enough, I was able to produce several compounds that would activate both receptors. I was excited. This was only a proof of concept but showed enormous potential.

Imagine an antiviral drug that became ineffective against a new mutant strain of a virus (as in the case of, for example, drugs targeting the HIV virus that causes AIDS). A drug designed in this way that loses its activity due to a change in the geometry of the ligand's active site could then twist around and bind to the altered active site of the mutant virus and keep its effectiveness, provided the altered site is still active (which can be easily tested). There are many potential applications for such drugs that could be effective against multiple variants of a virus or bacteria. An obvious one is a pandemic like Covid-19, where the virus keeps mutating into occasionally more dangerous or more infectious variants. If the treatments developed to deal with an earlier variant continued to work against a new variant, we could avoid or at least minimize recurrence of the disease.

My four-month license expired, and I postponed completing the project indefinitely. But I allowed myself to imagine how wonderful it could have been if I had completed the research and published the results in a journal with a fun title like: "Outsmarting a virus?"

* * *

My life after fifty involved trying things that I had always wanted to do but for which I had never had the time or energy (or courage). For example, very uncharacteristic for me, I auditioned for an amateur theatre production for the first time. I performed terribly in the audition but scored a non-speaking backdrop position in the man chorus anyway. I enjoyed the performances, but when the run ended, I was done with it. It wasn't as fun as I had imagined, but I was glad I tried. Another checklist item done.

When I was in Ankara, trying to get my business going, Vicki was able to visit me for two weeks. We joined an organized tour of Cappadocia. We were traveling in a small bus with about twenty Turkish people in the group. The guide would provide rich and interesting information about the sites in Turkish and I would try to translate it to Vicki. We were sitting at the very front, and the guide would speak English with us during the breaks to accommodate any questions that Vicki had.

The tour was amazing. The Cappadocia area features fairy chimneys, underground cities, and residences and churches both carved into the mountains. It represents a unique historical and cultural heritage as an early Christian site. For example, when the Romans systematically destroyed Christian churches in the first century AD, most of the Christian artifacts in Cappadocia survived since they were hidden in the churches carved into the mountains.

After Vicki returned to California, we met several more times through Skype. After a while, it became obvious that our long-distance relationship was not working, and since my move to Turkey was permanent, we decided to end the relationship.

* * *

Backgammon kept me busy in Turkey after I joined a club in Ankara. This active club promoted backgammon with the doubling cube, just like in the US. Play with the doubling cube was starting to gain popularity in large backgammon clubs in Ankara and Istanbul. They referred to it as modern backgammon to differentiate it from the classical backgammon that had been played without the doubling cube in the Middle East for millennia. I started playing in the Ankara club's leagues and tournaments. I garnered small tournament wins every now and then. The club started to travel as a group to play in different cities. I played in a tournament in Cyprus but didn't do well. I did better in Istanbul where a partner and I won the doubles championship. While I'd been able to earn money from US backgammon tournaments, monetary awards weren't common in Turkey. Perhaps it was thought of as gambling if money was involved. Instead, the awards were tangible gifts. Our win in Istanbul supplied each of us a large flatscreen television set.

My best performance in Turkey was at the Mediterranean Open tournament in Antalya. A player from Georgia (the country, not the state) eliminated me from the main tournament in the fourth round. My partner and I did better in the doubles tournament as we made it to the semifinals. He and I did not always see eye to eye. Our conflicting evaluations strained the partnership. At a certain point when our opponents gained a commanding lead, my partner got upset and left the table. I assumed he had gone outside to smoke a cigarette, which he did regularly, but this time he never returned. His wife, however, stayed at the table watching in solidarity with our team. Somehow, I was able to turn the game around, and we won and made it to the finals, to be played the next afternoon.

The Georgian player who eliminated me from the open tournament in the fourth round won the open individual tournament. He was also the half of the other finalist team in the doubles' tournament. His partner was from Belgium. The final match was a close 11-point game. When the score was tied at 9-9, I wanted to turn the doubling cube early. At this point, owning the cube would not advantage the opponent. They wouldn't be able to turn it again because a two-point cube was already enough to decide the 11-point match currently at 9-9, no matter who won. But I expected my partner to object to the idea (as he had in a similar situation in an earlier game). So, when my partner took a cigarette break, I turned the cube. With the cube at two and the 9-9 score, this would be the last game of the match. We won the game and the championship. Our reward, apart from accolades and trophies, was a laptop computer that I used for several years, so it was well worth the effort.

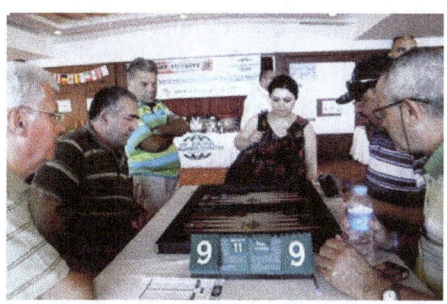

Mediterranean open doubles final game, I am on the right with black baseball cap

Meanwhile, while not generating contract-research work from Turkish pharmaceutical and bio-tech companies, Turkuaz Danış-manlık spurred me on to investigate opportunities for academic collaboration. A group at Hacettepe University was investigating phenylketonuria (PKU). In this rare but serious genetic disease, a misfolded phenylalanine hydroxylase enzyme disables the body's ability to break down phenylalanine. The normal enzyme manages the body's metabolism of phenylalanine, so people with this genetic disorder can't metabolize it. Found especially in protein-rich foods like meat, eggs, and dairy products, phenylalanine quickly reaches toxic levels in the blood of people with PKU.

Newborn babies are routinely evaluated for PKU, and those with the genetic disorder are subjected to a special diet, for life, that eliminates high-protein foods. Without treatment, PKU can damage the brain permanently and result in an irreversibly lowered IQ, learning disabilities, and other cognitive issues.

Worldwide, on average, 6.67 per 100,000 individuals have PKU. The lowest prevalence is in Finland (0.50 per 100,000), and the highest in

Turkey (38.46 per 100,000) based on available statistics at the time of this writing. Turkey had a clear reason to welcome and prioritize new treatments for PKU.

The Hacettepe University group and I together submitted a three-year research proposal to the Turkish Scientific and Technical Research Council (TUBITAK) to produce a drug-based treatment of PKU. The Hacettepe team identified a way to assess in a laboratory setting whether phenylalanine metabolism was functioning so they could test the biological activity of the new leads that I would propose. In return for a small commission to Turkuaz Danışmanlık, I would find these new biologically active small molecules (called chaperon ligands) with potential to repair the phenylalanine hydroxylase enzyme by helping the misfolded enzyme to fold properly. This low-cost project offered a potentially high return of treatment for a medical condition prevalent in Turkey; a project that I thought TUBITAK could not possibly reject. I was so sure the proposal would be funded that when it was not, I was stunned. This was the tipping point. Not a single contract in twelve months was enough for me.

I shut down the consulting business over three months and looked for something else to do. It was done. I was unemployed, once again. This would be the second time I entertained the idea of an early retirement.

* * *

Now that I had free time again, I scheduled some cruises as a bridge director. I wasn't being paid but, as a guest lecturer, did receive free cruises with one allowed guest. On one cruise, I invited a friend, Sevilla, who was a good bridge player and ran a bridge club in Encinitas, just north of San Diego. She had been my first girlfriend for six months following my divorce, and we remained good friends. During the cruise, she liked my bridge lessons and asked if I would give these lessons at her club and help her run some of her bridge games there. Considering that I had nothing much else to do, I accepted. She suggested that I could stay in her house and receive a percentage of the income for running the bridge games. She was generous, allowing me to keep all the income from the bridge classes I would teach. So, I temporarily moved back to the US.

In Encinitas, near San Diego again, I spent the next four months helping Sevilla run her bridge club and teaching bridge classes. One of the regular players in Sevilla's club had been a bridge student of mine five or six years earlier. Both she and her daughter took one of my beginning-bridge classes when I was teaching at Adventures in Bridge before my move to Turkey. Her daughter was married to the chief executive officer of the US subsidiary of a Japanese pharmaceutical company. I thought I might have a final shot at a pharmaceutical job if she could help. She suggested that I write a short proposal that she could send to her son-in-law. Apparently, he was busy, but he would have some time to read my proposal during his long flights to and from Japan.

My proposal detailed my offer. I would set up a computational facility requiring such-and-such hardware and software. With it up and running, I could discover new leads in therapeutic categories of interest to them. I offered to work for free during the first three months toward specific goals. If afterwards they agreed I had met the goals, I would become a regular employee. Knowing how difficult it was for a fifty-six-year-old person to get a job, I was offering free work as a hook. When I heard back from my student, her son-in-law didn't share my enthusiasm. He suggested that I apply for an open position in their Information Technology (IT) department.

When I say it was hard to find a job, I specifically mean a job where I could make an impact, make the world a better place. A job in the IT department is perfectly respectable. But I hoped to use my unique skills to make important contributions to medical science. These types of jobs *were* difficult to get. And while every company claims they do not discriminate based on age, from my perspective it felt like a consideration in employment decisions. In my life after fifty I found it difficult to gain new employment.

About this time, I got an email from my old friend, Phil Bowen, checking up on me and updating me on his life. He had moved to a small private university in Atlanta, Georgia and got approval and funding to start a "Center for Drug Design." He asked if I could help him get the Center started. I agreed to join him as a research associate for a few years to help him with the Center and perform some drug design projects. This latter possibility was attractive to me. Finally, I would be involved in discovery of new, biologically active chemical entities, like the work I did at J&J, but not proprietary, so we could publish the results.

After four months at Encinitas, I returned to Turkey. The job in Atlanta would be a part-time, four-days-a-week work, 80% of a full-time job. It was essentially my second post-doctoral appointment some twenty years after my first. Soon after, Phil got the paperwork completed and sent me the job offer. And I was on my way back to the US again.

# CHAPTER 11

# At Mercer University

*Atlanta, Georgia, 2012-2015*

I landed in Atlanta mid-August 2012 with only two suitcases in my possession. I rented a small, furnished apartment about a mile from the campus of Mercer University and settled in. Mercer is a small private college with its main campus in Macon, Georgia. The Atlanta campus, with the Pharmacy Department and Phil, is relatively small and hosts a few departments of the graduate school.

Monday morning, I walked the mile to the Atlanta campus from my apartment. It was humid and hot. Heat I can deal with, but humidity is a different story. I was soaking wet when I made it to the campus. What a way to make a first impression! Since Phil was out of town, I needed to find the Human Resources (HR) department. My contact in HR wanted to see my visa but, when he saw that I had an American passport, the process got easier. After completing the paperwork, he gave me my keys and took me over to where the Center for Drug Design would be set up. The place was packed with boxes. With a little effort, I cleaned up a desk for my laptop and worked on the multitude of little tasks (like getting an email account) to set myself up in the Mercer network.

Wanting to help me to get started in Atlanta, Vicki visited me over Labor Day weekend. We drove around with her rental car and shopped for all the things I needed and ran errands that I couldn't otherwise do because I didn't have a car yet. I appreciated Vicki's thoughtfulness.

Eventually all the boxes in the lab got moved out, and I could move around and get the infrastructure work started. The computational research lab was going to have different electrical lines than the rest of the building. We set up three cubicles as workspaces for three people and a general work area for the big computer (i.e., our private server). Each work area would have a beefed-up PC. The large color printer sat next to the computer server. Phil framed several colored screen shots of various molecular models. Arranged nicely on the walls, they helped the room start to resemble a presentable computer lab. I contacted the software company (Schrödinger) for their system requirements incorporating all the tools I would need for small-molecule modeling, some applications for macromolecular modeling, and the *Phase* application for pharmacophore model generation. Our main server would have 32 central processing units (making it powerful) and a large amount of memory (making it fast) and several large hard drives on which I could construct databases. When it arrived in the lab, we connected it to the network, and it was ready to go. We also installed large storage batteries to keep the system going uninterrupted for some time in case of a power outage.

The hardware for the computational chemistry lab was ready. Acquiring the needed software (the cost of which was significantly higher than that of the hardware) took some creativity. With no immediate budget available, I contacted the software company and arranged for a four-month evaluation license for all the applications I wanted to use. Once installed, we could test and set up the software environment and I could start some of the work while budget negotiations continued.

For any productive work in pharmacophore modeling, we needed three-dimensional (3D) structural databases. We ordered a database of commercial products, but it was not useful other than serving as a good starting point. I needed to start building the databases that I wanted right away. When using predictive models, the higher quality the databases, the higher quality the results.[22] I downloaded the Structure/data file (SD file) of the publicly available Sigma/Aldrich chemicals catalog and started building it in *Phase* format to set up and evaluate the process. I planned to build in the future other structural databases for chemicals of interest, including existing drugs on the market, potential future drugs in development, and other chemicals in commercial chemicals catalogs and published databases of known chemicals. I prioritized all of these to convert into a format that I could use with *Phase*. This database-building work started at once and continued in parallel to other work we did for the duration of my stay in Atlanta. By the time I was finishing at Mercer, two and a half years later, we had built a series of databases of over eight million compounds.

While we were getting things going in the lab, I took a week's break and visited Vicki in California. It was fun to visit the sites that we had frequented a couple of years back and reminisce about the good old days. This also gave us a chance to reevaluate our relationship. In the end, we decided that, even though we were only two time zones away from each other as opposed to the ten when I lived in Turkey, it was still a long-distance relationship that was not working. Really, though, I think I was "damaged goods" by that time. After having worked so hard and for so long to get a divorce, I couldn't get myself to commit to further this relationship. This would be our final breakup.

* * *

Phil and I started interviewing the Mercer faculty to evaluate collaboration opportunities. Once the lab was fully up and running, we intended to expand the collaborations to external universities as well, per the goals and aims of the Center for Drug Design. Meanwhile, to evaluate the system and work out any kinks, I needed a small project to complete in the four-month window of our free license. One of the scientists at Mercer was working on paralytic shellfish poisoning (PSP). She was enthusiastic about collaborating with us. PSP occurs when people ingest shellfish, usually clams and oysters, that have absorbed toxins from the algae that the shellfish had ingested as food. People who ingest high levels of the toxin can suffer serious illness and even die. So our first project sought a drug-based treatment for paralytic shellfish poisoning.

I gathered the structures of all the known chemicals that contribute to PSP and started developing pharmacophore models. The experimental team was not ready to assess new chemicals, so I used the time to figure out which models were selective to the known poisons. I built a small decoy database and seeded it with the known poisons and used the multitude of pharmacophore models that I had developed to search this database. I evaluated the results for candidate compounds, using the GH-Score Dr. Henry and I had developed at Molecular Design Limited. I subjected each pharmacophore model to rigorous analysis and prioritized the hit lists based on their GH-Score and other considerations. Once I found the best models, I ran them on some of the databases of commercially available chemicals and, after carefully prioritizing them, I proposed to the experimental team several chemicals for them to buy and test. Meanwhile the evaluation license expired, and we still did not have the budget to license the software systems.

The "paralytic" in PSP is because the toxin involved causes paralysis of the upper respiratory system. It does this by blocking sodium channels, which are like flippable switches in excitable cells such as muscle cells and neurons. We sought a small-molecule drug to swap out the toxin blocking the channel, which would allow the switch to work again. Physicians use a similar concept to treat methanol poisoning. They provide the patient with a large amount of ethanol (e.g., absolute vodka). The ethanol molecules swap with the methanol, which is then excreted from the body.

So to find an appropriate molecule to treat PSP, we had to show that the candidate drug molecule blocked inhibition of the sodium channels, but we encountered a problem. Apparently, the way the experimental team was testing the chemicals was incompatible with the way we had modeled how these chemicals would bind to a receptor site and cause a biologically significant reaction. To grossly oversimplify, it was like training a monkey to recognize the difference between plums and apricots and then testing them with plumcots. I was disappointed that we had not communicated well with the experimental team, and specifically that we did not have a way to test for enzyme inhibition.

For future collaborations, we would clarify the roles of each team member before starting work. But for now, since the experimental team was not able to assess the biological activity of the proposed compounds, the project could not continue. I was frustrated that my four months of hard work on our first project was wasted. But at least it allowed us to get the system running and got some small databases built during the software evaluation period.

We kept busy while waiting for the budget approval. Phil had made a commitment to write a review article on a framework for predicting aspects of toxicity (ADME/Tox, where ADME stand for adsorption, distribution, metabolism and excretion) for the *Current Topics in Medicinal Chemistry* journal. Once we started the work, we decided to split the papers in two, where Phil would author the paper from a quantum mechanical perspective,[23] and I would write the review from a pharmacophore modeling perspective.[24]

One of my checklist items was to investigate the origin of the pharmacophore concept. Since pharmacophore modeling was my area of expertise, I felt I should be involved with addressing the conflicting claims in the literature about its origins and perhaps even try to resolve the conflict. I had wanted to work on this for some time , but I had little access to published literature as a civilian. Such a project meant reviewing hundreds of scientific papers, some of which would be over a century old. I couldn't afford the $25 to $50 per paper an individual would be charged. However, as an employee of a university with a broad license to most journals, I could download and review these papers for free. Most of the searches were online, and most of the time, I would need to use the Interlibrary Loan system to get the electronic versions of the papers I needed.

This was excellent. While the infrastructure work was slowly moving ahead, Phil and I were able to use the time to write a scientific detective study to resolve the conflict over the origin of the pharmacophore concept. It took us about a year to complete, but we got it done, and the paper was published.[25] We demonstrated that Dr. Paul Ehrlich (recipient of the Nobel Prize in medicine, 1908) originated the concept in 1898. Though he had clearly originated the concept, Dr. Ehrlich had never used the term pharmacophore in any of his papers. He used the term toxophores, while his contemporaries referred to pharmacophores, leading to much of the confusion that our paper cleared up. Perhaps Dr. Ehrlich did not appreciate someone else naming his baby.[26] When I consider all the papers I have published, this is the one in which I take the most pride.

* * *

After graduating from Connecticut College with a degree in international relations and an anthropology minor, Sibel moved to Washington DC to start a career in international relations. She took a job as a server in a posh Italian restaurant in DuPont Circle while searching for an internship. She eventually got a receptionist job, but she wasn't happy being in DC.

She had heard from me about my amazing college years, with friendships enduring difficult circumstances. She knew that despite the hardships, those were my most memorable days, and those friendships were for life. Sibel never had that opportunity during college. She transferred out of Boston College after her first year to Connecticut College for a year, then moved to Italy for a semester before returning to finish her degree in Connecticut. She moved around, took extra classes, and worked full-time throughout college, making her too busy to focus on her social network and preventing her from establishing long-term friendships. This, she said, was missing in her life: a good college life with deep friendships. So she decided to go back to school for a master's degree. She wanted to pursue a master's in social sciences at a university with a strong international focus. She identified a half dozen programs in the US and one in Germany. She applied for the Global Studies Program at the University of Freiburg and got accepted even before she had a chance to apply for any of the universities in the US.

Apart from a rewarding university life, the global studies program provided Sibel opportunities to travel around the world and experience different cultures. The master's program was centered at the University of Freiburg in Germany. After finishing the first semester in Germany, she would take the second semester at Cape Town University in South Africa and the third semester in the Jawaharlal Nehru University (JNU) in New Delhi, India. Then she would do a three-month summer internship somewhere in the world, and finish with her last semester back in Freiburg. She loved the opportunity to study in different universities in different continents and to immerse herself in different cultures. For me, it was great to see her so excited and happy again.

\* \* \*

Our budget finally came through and we received a three-year license on the software packages that we asked for. Because we had had the opportunity to set up the system and get trained on various applications during the evaluation period, we hit the ground running. At any given point, we were working on two (or sometimes even three) different projects simultaneously. They would each be in various stages so did not compete for the same resources. I supply here a synopsis of four projects that resulted in publications to showcase the diversity of the work we conducted at the Center for Drug Design at Mercer University.

\* \* \*

## Nonpsychedelic serotonin agonists - for potential treatment of depression

This internal project at Mercer University looked at serotonin 2A (5-HT$_{2A}$) receptor agonists. Some existing medications to treat depression focus on the availability of the neurotransmitter serotonin to facilitate the firing of certain kinds of brain cells by either making more serotonin available or allowing what is produced to stick around longer for more effect, making them serotonin "agonists." Some psychedelic compounds that work in one of these ways have been found to be effective against depression—with the drawback that they are psychedelic. The goal, therefore, would be to find or produce a compound that has the desirable curative effect without the undesirable hallucinatory effect.

We thought we could develop a pharmacophore model that differentiates serotonin agonists with and without psychedelic effects. Then we would use the model to search and retrieve new compounds that could potentially be used therapeutically. We started with the evaluation of two compounds: non-psychedelic 5-HT$_{2A}$ receptor agonist lisuride, and psychedelic 5-HT$_{2A}$ receptor agonist lysergic acid diethylamide (LSD).

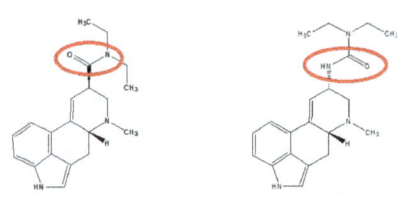

LSD on the left and Lisuride on the right; highlighted area shows the small structural difference with large therapeutic effect

The exceedingly small structural difference between these two compounds is in the position of the amide group (highlighted with red ellipses in the figure). Both compounds are serotonin agonists; however, LSD is hallucinogenic, while lisuride is not. As a drug, lisuride (Dopergin®), is mainly used to treat migraines because it is also a dopamine agonist and has recently been considered to treat Parkinson's disease as well. It was not approved by the US Food and Drug Administration but had been on the market in some other countries. Our interest in lisuride for this project was merely due to its structural similarity to LSD without the psychedelic side effect. With these characteristics, lisuride would be an ideal compound on which to base the project's first pharmacophore model. Evaluating it together with LSD, we hoped to find a differentiating feature.

We developed a pharmacophore model using the structure of lisuride. When we flexibly aligned both lisuride and LSD with the pharmacophore model, an interesting picture appeared. While lisuride managed to match all the features of the pharmacophore model (obviously since the model was developed based on it), LSD could not match the hydrogen-bond acceptor site (pink in the figure), while it did match all the other features.

By using this pharmacophore model, we searched various structural databases and scrutinized the hit lists to make sure that the compounds strongly matched the pharmacophore model. Importantly, they had to match the H-bond acceptor site that seems to block the psychedelic effect (the feature that LSD could not fit). When we searched the database of known drugs, we retrieved some compounds as potential serotonin agonists without the hallucinogenic side-effect.

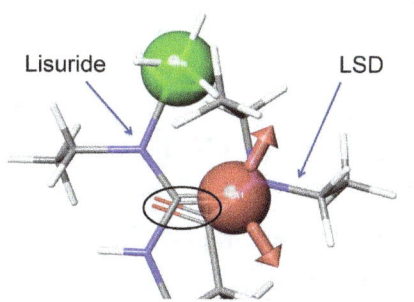

**Highlighted with black ellipse, the figure shows the carbonyl oxygen of LSD pointing in the opposite direction and missing the pink colored H-bond acceptor site.**
*Reprinted with permission from reference 27. Copyright © 2019 Elsevier Inc.*

A beta blocker used to treat heart failure and high blood pressure; carvedilol was one of the compounds retrieved with this model. We decided to pursue biological testing of this compound, since it was an existing drug that scientists could repurpose. If it were indeed found to be a serotonin agonist without the hallucinogenic side effect, it could potentially treat depression, addiction recovery, or other serotonin-related conditions. Repurposing is attractive in drug design because, unlike a new chemical entity, the compound has already gone through rigorous safety assessments, saving significant development costs compared to an untested candidate.

Our co-workers verified the serotonin agonist activity of carvedilol. They also verified that it did not induce a hallucinogenic effect. We did not pursue intellectual property protection (i.e., a patent) for this study. Instead, we decided to put the study in the public domain, and we published the computational and experimental details of this work.[27] Pharmaceutical serotonin agonists could potentially be used to treat the following medical conditions:

- Migraine headache
- Depression

- Anxiety
- Schizophrenia
- Drug addiction

* * *

## AKT inhibitors study – for potential treatment of cancer

P13K/AKT is a growth-regulating molecular pathway that is over-activated in many human cancers.[28] AKT is an enzyme in that pathway. A type of drug candidate called AKT inhibitors had been shown to decrease the phosphorylation of AKT.[29] This decrease in phosphorylation had been associated with a reduction in tumor cell proliferation. Our aim was to produce a new class of AKT inhibitors with potentially better attributes than those in development elsewhere.

One known inhibitor of AKT was the natural chemical solenopsin, from venom excreted by the red fire ant. We developed a pharmacophore model based on the structure of solenopsin then compared thousands of compounds in the database to it. The study retrieved many steroids, which matched the model but did not fit other criteria, like molecule size. However, among smaller-sized compounds in the hit list were several compounds that structurally resembled solenopsin, three of which were biologically tested.

**Solenopsin**

Each compound has a long carbon side chain on either a heterocyclic ring system or equivalent open chain functional group. Biological laboratory testing confirmed that all three were AKT pathway inhibitors. These laboratory experiments showed that the second compound significantly inhibited proliferation of a specific type of lung carcinoma (a type of cancer) cells called H2009.[30] A small dose of this compound provided a reasonable level of biological effect, suggesting it as a potential drug candidate. We published details of the study;[31] followed by a review article.[32]

Patients with the following types of cancers could potentially benefit from such treatment:

- Lung
- Breast
- Ovarian
- Prostate
- Bladder
- Colorectal

\* \* \*

## Potential treatment for neurodegenerative diseases – Alzheimer's, Parkinson's, and Huntington's

As the Center gained more experience and credibility, we started to collaborate with external universities to take advantage of each other's complementary strengths. In this project, we collaborated with a group from the University of Georgia.

The kynurenine molecular pathway had been discovered to play a key role in many neurodegenerative diseases. It is a major route for the catabolism (breakdown) of tryptophan. In this pathway, the kynurenine monooxygenase enzyme (KMO) is of particular interest because as it does its work it produces toxic molecules. The final compound in the pathway, quinolinic acid (QUIN), is neurotoxic. But the compound before the KMO enzyme reaction, kynurenine (KYNA), is neuro protective. The ratio of KYNA to QUIN is considered an important measurement since it is favorable (more KYNA) to neuroprotection in healthy individuals and unfavorable (more QUIN) in people afflicted with neurodegenerative diseases.

KYNA

KMO

L-tryptophan

UPF 648

Quinolinic acid
QUIN

**Part of the tryptophan metabolism that involves KMO enzyme inhibition**

A compound that inhibits KMO may moderate the formation of neurotoxic QUIN and increase the KYNA/QUIN ratio. One compound, UPF 648, is an extensively studied inhibitor of KMO. However, UPF 648 has unfavorable side effects that make it unsuitable as a drug. It increases the production of hydrogen peroxide twenty-fold, resulting in harmful *oxidative stress* (see next example). Nevertheless, UPF 648 served as an important model in developing KMO inhibitors since the easily obtained yeast-KMO with UPF 648 is identical to human KMO. By using the bound conformation of UPF 648, we developed a pharmacophore model with which we retrieved several potential inhibitors. Appendix I details the steps we took to develop the pharmacophore model and retrieve new active compounds.

Neurotoxicity from a low KYNA/QUIN ratio occurs in the three neurodegenerative diseases named after their discoverers, Huntington's, Alzheimer's, and Parkinson's, as well as the following medical conditions:

- Epilepsy
- Neuropsychiatric disorders
- Stroke
- Other immune-related diseases

A new drug that can moderate the metabolism of tryptophan through inhibition of KMO could potentially offer a treatment for these conditions. We published the details of the discovery of the active molecules and their biological testing results.[33] My colleagues and I followed up with comprehensive information pertaining to KMO inhibitors in a recent review article.[34]

* * *

## *Potential treatment for oxidative stress*

This research involved a collaboration among four universities. We at Mercer identified new chemical entities. The cardiology group at Emory University conducted biological testing. The team at Union University in Tennessee synthesized analogs (comparable molecules) of the lead compounds. And finally, the team from Howard University took part in a second iteration of molecular modeling and analysis.

Oxidative stress plays a fundamental role in many disease states. Cells naturally produce two opposing kinds of molecules while functioning: free radicals and antioxidants. Free radicals are molecules with an unpaired electron that can bind easily with other molecules—like DNA—in the cell, with a destructive result. Antioxidants can bind with the free radicals and take them out of action. Oxidative stress occurs when there is a massive imbalance in the ratio of free radicals (and an associated reactive oxygen species called ROS) to antioxidants. The excessive production of these radicals and ROSs is linked to many inflammatory diseases like heart disease, arthritis, and diabetes.

To help protect the body from pathogens, Nox enzymes, including Nox4, produce hydrogen peroxide, an ROS. While hydrogen peroxide helps fight pathogens, it can also be noxious to human cells when not properly moderated by other molecules in the body. Our interest was to investigate new chemical entities that could moderate free radicals to reduce Nox4's release of hydrogen peroxide ($H_2O_2$) into the bloodstream.

Unlike the study above (KMO inhibitors) where we had access to a 3D structure of the target enzyme bound with a ligand and were able to use the 3D structure of the bound ligand to build the pharmacophore models, we did not have this opportunity with the Nox4 inhibitors project. We had to develop the pharmacophore models by finding the common patterns of known active compounds.

Appendix II provides details of how we generated the pharmacophore model and retrieved active compounds. We published how we optimized the lead molecules from among the active compounds we found.[35] And we followed up with a review article.[36] In this case, we also sought intellectual property protection.[37]

If our lead compound eventually became a drug for treatment of oxidative stress, it could potentially be used for the treatment of, for example, the following medical conditions:

- Kidney and lung fibrosis
- Cell proliferation in cancer
- Brain damage after stroke
- Cardiac hypertrophy and contractile dysfunction
- Diabetic nephropathy
- Arthritis
- Osteoporosis
- Peripheral nerve injury
- Atherosclerosis
- Restenosis after angioplasty
- Aneurisms
- Pulmonary hypertension
- Leprechaunism

A drug that inhibits Nox4 would offer a good example of the concept of treating the underlying disease, not just the medical signs or symptoms of a disease. For example, medications like antiacids treat the symptom, upset stomach from excess stomach acid. The drug can relieve the symptoms, and even neutralize the stomach acids that caused those symptoms, but it does nothing to address the true underlying cause of the excess stomach acids, which may be, for example, an ulcer, itself caused by a bacterial infection. In this instance, a treatment for the underlying cause, an antibiotic regimen, can cure the disease and eliminate the symptoms altogether. Similarly, antihypertensive medications to reduce blood pressure, statins to reduce cholesterol levels, pain killers to reduce pain, all address medical signs (high blood pressure, elevated cholesterol) or symptoms (pain) of these diseases, but most of them do not get at the underlying cause of these signs and symptoms.

Likewise, when Nox enzymes release excess hydrogen peroxide and cause oxidative stress leading to symptoms such as fatigue, memory loss, and brain fog, doctors can prescribe antioxidants to react with and neutralize the hydrogen peroxide in an effort to eliminate the symptoms. This approach only targets the medical sign (elevated hydrogen peroxide) and symptoms of oxidative stress. It also requires an impractically large dose and does not work very well. However, a drug to inhibit Nox4 would get at the underlying biochemical mechanism and reduce the release of hydrogen peroxide in the first place, preventing oxidative stress and eliminating the need to take antioxidants. It would treat the actual disease.

\* \* \*

The Atlanta campus of Mercer university had a spectacular nature trail that I explored almost daily during my lunch hours. The hilly two and a half miles through thick forest gave me a good cardiovascular workout. After strong storms, fallen trees would block trails and temporarily close the route. I'd eagerly await its reopening because access to this beautiful natural area provided some of my most pleasurable moments in Atlanta.

Meanwhile, every time I drove by the salsa club close to the Mercer University campus, I considered whether it was time to learn salsa. I procrastinated while trying to gather enough courage to join the salsa club, right until my time in Atlanta ended.

\* \* \*

I spent two and a half productive years in Atlanta. Except for the first failed project (paralytic shellfish poisoning), all the other projects yielded biologically active novel compounds. After burning out at Accelrys, I wanted to do only things I enjoyed. And, since I started my consulting business, I wanted to try to design new drugs, something I knew I would enjoy, and did. When I finished my term at Mercer, I could check this important item off my list.

Having done so, I gave myself permission to again consider opportunities at software companies for potential employment—but only opportunities that I would enjoy.

# CHAPTER 12

# World Cruise

*Burlingame, California, 2015-2016*

At the end of my term at Mercer University, a small software company in Burlingame, California recruited me to start in April of 2015. They wanted me to launch their marketing organization. I was excited to have a full-time job. Unfortunately, it did not last long as I did not see eye to eye with the chief executive officer. I felt like I was given responsibility without the needed authority. When I work in a supportive environment, I perform well. When I work in a non-supportive environment, however, I perform poorly. So, things were not going well at work. When I turned 59 and a half, I resigned, four months after my start.

At this age, I could withdraw from my retirement account (a rollover IRA) without an early withdrawal penalty. Despite a financially humble start to my professional life in the US, I was able to secure a plain retirement for myself. I could pay myself a salary until I figured out what to do with my semi-retirement, again.

\* \* \*

Burlingame was one of the more expensive cities in the Bay Area. I didn't want to burn through my retirement funds too rapidly. To make ends meet, I needed to make money to offset excess costs. Then I remembered my high school organic chemistry teacher, Vitali Meşulam, who had inspired me to become a chemist.

As I considered my post-retirement work options, I thought it might be my turn to inspire the next generations into science. I decided to teach chemistry, but at what level? Elementary, middle, or high school? College level? I visited several schools in the area and quickly decided that I could not teach kindergarten to twelfth grade. I would need to develop specific skills to teach kids. Up to this point, all my teaching experience was with adults. So, I quickly focused on college-level opportunities. To have more impact with my inspirational aspiration, I would teach introductory-level courses like general chemistry, perhaps in community colleges.

Meanwhile, because I was unemployed, I had time to take on longer cruises as a bridge director. I jumped at one such opportunity, a cruise circumnavigating the globe, to start on January 20, 2016. I had dreamed of doing a world cruise for a long time but could never afford the time off, almost four months, when I was employed. I remember browsing through the itinerary of various world cruises trying to imagine all the shore excursions I could do at each stop. Now I could check another big item off on my bucket list.

I had just over three months to prepare for this long voyage and at the same time to start applying for part-time teaching jobs in nearby community colleges. I didn't want to be stuck at home doing these applications, so I went to do my work at the Burlingame Public Library as if I were going to my office each day. This also gave me an opportunity to walk the mile to and from the library, and once again include exercise in my routine.

Preparing the documents for each job application took time and consideration. I committed one to two library hours to this task every day until the cruise and in that time applied to seven or eight nearby community colleges for part-time teaching positions. One of the positions was a bit far afield, about fifty-five miles north of San Francisco in Santa Rosa. I initially dismissed it since it would be a two-hour oneway commute over the crowded Golden Gate Bridge from Burlingame.

At the last minute, I did apply for it; I had the documents prepared already, so what could I lose? The applications would take several months to process, by which time I'd be back from my cruise. So the timing worked out nicely.

\* \* \*

Kurt was still working on his PhD in history at the University of Utah, but also worked several jobs, including teaching at community colleges. His PhD dissertation work took a back seat when he got a full-time job managing the education and curriculum in Utah's state prison system—a program that he designed and pitched himself. He and his fiancé, Emily, decided to get married in October 2016. My mom and my sister Mine and her husband Demir flew in a month before the wedding to do some sightseeing in San Francisco. Mine and Demir leased an apartment in the Haight-Ashbury district, of 1960s hippie fame. Mom stayed with me in Burlingame. Once Mine and Demir got San Francisco out of their system, we all rented a car to drive to Salt Lake City. The beautifully organized wedding took place at the Tracy Aviary, with birds large and small providing a visual and musical backdrop. One of Kurt's friends officiated the ceremony, another provided live music, and one of his former students tended the bar; Emily's grandmother handled the flower arrangements, her mom made her dress, and her best friend designed the invitations; and Sibel contributed by designing the tables' place cards. A few people spoke, reminiscing and engendering some tears.

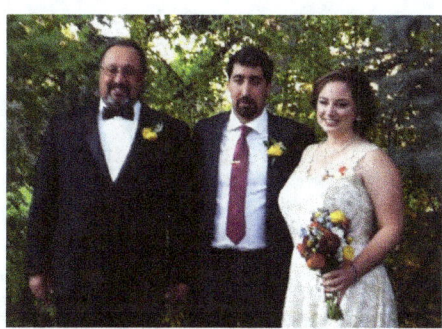

At Emily and Kurt's wedding

After the official wedding ceremony, a large outdoor buffet served up delicious Mediterranean food, with a nice Turkish menu introducing attendees to the cuisine's charms. We joyously celebrated with most of our core family there: Mom, Mine and Demir came from Turkey; Sibel came from South Africa; and I from California. We mingled during dinner with Emily's extended family, who came from all around the US, and other fun guests. I was happy to meet some of Kurt's professors and his friends. After dinner we all moved to the indoor reception, where Kurt and Emily's friends reminisced about some of their shared memories with the two. Nice music, dancing, the wedding cake. Everyone was happy.

Mom was tired and wanted to leave a little early. She, Mine and Demir went to their car and waited for Sibel and me. It took us close to half an hour to say all our goodbyes. I felt guilty for keeping them waiting in the car; and I also felt guilty for having to leave the reception early. Our fellow travelers were patient and we eventually made it back to our hotel rooms. The next day we drove back to Burlingame, and shortly after Mom, Mine, and Demir returned to Turkey.

* * *

Back in Burlingame, it was time for me to prepare for the long cruise. My bridge contributions on these trips were needed only on at-sea days. When the ship was docked in port, I would be free to do whatever I wanted—stroll through the town, take an organized tour offered by the cruise ship, or even just relax onboard. The nearly four-month cruise had seventy at-sea days during which I would teach one-hour classes in the mornings and run sanctioned games in the afternoons, where the participants could earn American Contract Bridge League master-points. I would need to prepare at least seventy bridge lectures. (I ended up with 71 lectures because I decided to teach during the crossing of the Suez Canal – not technically an at-sea day, but a cool time to lecture about bridge!)

Assuming that most passengers would be taking the whole trip, I could develop a progressive series of classes allowing the participants to advance gradually in their mastery of bridge. I labeled the clusters of classes as Bridge 101, 102, Bridge 201, and so forth, much like college courses. This way, someone who had never played bridge before could start learning to play with Bridge 101, and several months later, after finishing Bridge 401, could "graduate" from the program as a proper duplicate bridge player.[38] And they would achieve all this during a long cruise circling the globe. They would have developed the skills to play at their local clubs back home and hold their own against more experienced players. On the cruise they could also earn masterpoints by playing at the sanctioned afternoon bridge games.

I had always gone above and beyond what was required for the bridge program on cruise ships, though I don't think the cruise directors ever noticed. As far as they were concerned, I was just another bridge director, and we all did the same thing.

For example, before I came aboard, I would run a software application to set up pre-dealt hands, provide a computer analysis of the hands for each game, and bring the printed results with me on the ship. At the end of each game, players would record their results on a "traveler," a score pad that remained with a duplicate board where every team, after playing the hands, would score their results. Then they could see the analyses I brought and find out what would have been possible if they had performed the best play.

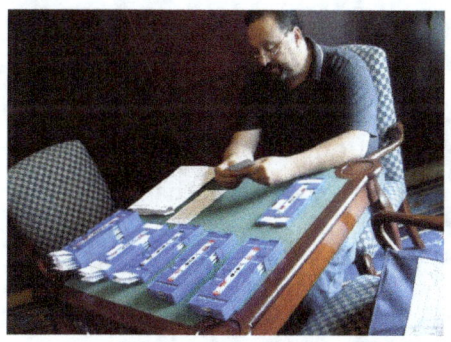

Preparing the duplicate bridge boards for the next day's game

While players appreciated this opportunity, it was a lot of extra work for me. Every night before the next day's game, I would spend over an hour setting up all the duplicate boards to match the pre-dealt hands for which I had analyses. To my knowledge, no other director took this level of care on cruise ships. They would simply have the players shuffle and deal during the first round and everyone else would play those same boards the remaining rounds. Even if the ship administrators didn't notice this extra effort, I had set a high standard for myself, and I felt better upholding it.

Comparing identical hands with identical decks in duplicate bridge games is the standard competitive game. For the world cruise though, with so many games, the weight and volume of the paper needed for my analyses would have taken all my luggage space, space that I could not afford to waste. Regardless of how long or short the cruise, I still have a fifty-pound luggage limit when flying to the embarkation port. So, for this cruise, I did what all the other bridge directors do; have the players shuffle and deal the boards in the first round.

Even with that decision, it took creativity to stay within the luggage space and weight limit for this extensive voyage. The first stop after sailing from Los Angeles was in Honolulu, Hawaii. I knew that the cruise ship port was two blocks from downtown Honolulu with several large stores like Walmart and Ross. So I decided to buy some of the needed clothing and incidentals there instead of loading them in my luggage for the flight to Los Angeles, where I would finally board the Pacific Princess®.

The boat's name may be familiar to people who remember an old sitcom called *The Love Boat*. (A channel on the ship's internal television system was dedicated to reruns of the show.) This small cruise ship had a maximum capacity of six-hundred-and-forty passengers and was way more fun than an old sitcom. See Appendix V for the trip's itinerary.

* * *

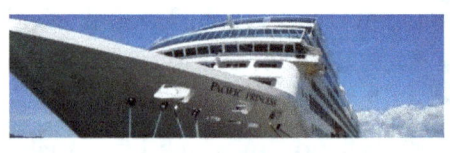

Pacific Princess®

Midnight on February 1, 2016 came to us later than anywhere else in the world as we crossed the international date line. Early the next morning, I was exercise-walking on the ship's top level. I caught the rising sun, and I was probably the one of the very first people (in the entire world) to see the sun rise that day. The ship's captain and crew were on a lower deck, so I saw the morning sun even before they did. It was the morning of February 3, because we skipped February 2 while crossing the international date line.

Because of the westward movement of the ship, each day on board was slightly longer than twenty-four hours. These extra minutes added up to exactly twenty-four hours by the end of the cruise. At the end of the 111th day on the cruise ship, 112 days had passed in Los Angeles. The missing day, February 2, 2016, didn't exist for us.

This gave me more appreciation for Jules Verne's classic novel *Around the World in 80 Days*. The protagonists were moving eastward (opposite to us) and, at the end of their trip, they had under their belts an extra day of which they weren't aware. They thought that they lost by one day their bet to circle the globe in 80 days, but later learned that they had won. I had been intrigued by this phenomenon, and now I had experienced it in reverse.

About two thirds of the participants in the bridge program were making the full circumnavigation and could take full advantage of my progressive bridge classes. The other third would take one of the six segments of the cruise. I enjoyed the typical benefits of a cruise ship where the cabins were cleaned twice every day, gourmet food was available for lunch and dinner, and room service promised food twenty-four hours a day. Broadway style shows played every night, and we visited some of the most exotic places in the world, all without changing accommodations. I could get used to this. What an excellent way to start my retirement! While at sea, the cruise director provided varied fun activities, like my bridge program. The engaging circumnavigating bridge group made my entire cruise enjoyable.

What kind of people take cruises? Is there a typical characteristic that defines regular cruise goers? A broad spectrum of people takes short cruises: young, old, party goers, families with children, retirees, single people, persons with disabilities. Specialized cruise businesses target different groups, for example, Disney (for families with children), Carnival (for younger/middle-aged groups), Holland American (for the elderly). On show themed cruises, like the *Prairie Home Companion* cruise, fans pay a small premium to join a cruise loaded with specific shows performed by their favorite entertainers. On bridge cruises, participants pay extra to compete in sectional or regional level tournaments on the cruise, with a choice of different levels of offered bridge classes. These differ from the bridge program that I administered, which is free and open to all guests, but only during at-sea days. Bridge-thematic cruises instead offer multiple daily bridge activities, even when in port. Once you take a cruise, on-board incentives entice you to book your next cruise before you depart. Once you have several cruises under your belt, you get discounts and other perks when you book again, similar to frequent flyer programs.

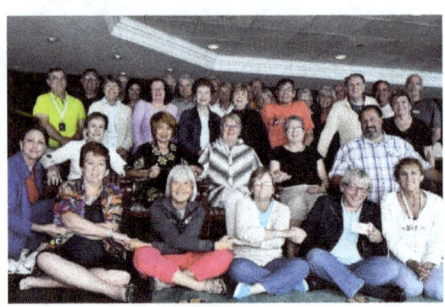

The bridge group on the world cruise. I am at the right end in the second row.

But who would take cruises of three or four weeks or longer? Or very long cruises like my world cruise? Only those with available time. Most working people don't have that much time, or if they do, they need to split their earned vacation days with other scheduled activities like family visits or time at time-shares. That leaves a narrow candidate profile: retired, wealthy individuals. You will find plenty of wealthy, widowed women and men. And very wealthy individuals who can afford to delegate someone to run their businesses while taking a long break. And then there are people using cruises as an alternative to retirement homes or assisted living. If they don't have a serious medical condition, the long cruises are a lot cheaper than nursing homes, and you get all the cruise perks.

My experience is that most of the people I see at the dinner table on these long cruises are wealthy, white, privileged, mostly conservative retired people. At least for American clientele. Europeans tend to have more vacation days, allowing for younger and more active cruisers on the longer cruises.

There are, of course, exceptions. On the world cruise, for example, an elder black lady joined our table for just one segment. She was a retired schoolteacher, and the cruise was a gift from her children upon her retirement. She was witty and a delightful conversationalist. We were typically the last two people at our dinner table. Her friends would stop by our table to chat and ask her if she would introduce her new boyfriend(!). Because she needed help walking, I would offer her my arm and we would walk all the way to her cabin before saying our goodbyes. At the end of that segment she left, and that was that.

Most people gain weight on short cruises because of the constant availability of good food. On long cruises, however, I find that it's possible to avoid gaining weight. After the third week, you've tried all of the dishes. You start developing routines, things get settled and perhaps you go back to your oatmeal breakfast and walking miles around the top deck. Not drinking alcohol certainly helps. If you like alcohol (which is abundantly available on every cruise ship), then all bets are off. You will likely finish the cruise barely fitting into the clothes that you came in with.

* * *

One morning as I sat watching the sun rise somewhere over the Atlantic Ocean, my mind wandered to the physics of the beautiful colors before me. Beyond appreciating the orange/red colors spread around the sun, I thought about the Tyndall effect: that what I was seeing was the particles in the air scattering high-energy light (blue-violet) away into the atmosphere allowing low-energy light (red-orange) to reach my eyes.

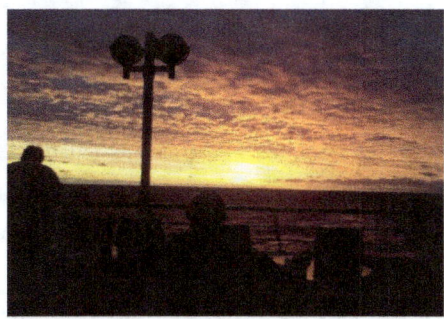

The veranda on the Pacific Princess®, where I had my early breakfasts while enjoying the sun rise.

The Tyndall effect is also what gives someone deep blue eyes. The blue eye color is not from pigmentation, but from particles that scatter and distribute the high-energy light, in this case back toward the viewer, similar to why our sky is blue.

I also enjoy seeing a full moon, but my thoughts wander at times to the mechanics of what I see. I think about the life span of a photon. A photon comes into being during the nuclear fusion reactions in the core of the sun as an extremely high energy gamma ray. With all the collisions it has to endure during its long trip to the surface of the sun, it progressively loses energy, with the gamma radiation reducing to X-ray and ultraviolet radiation, and eventually to visible light. It takes between half-a-million to a million years for a photon to make its way out to the surface of the sun and finally escape from it. Then another eight minutes to reach the moon. Finally, the reflected light from the moon takes about a second to reach our eyes. That is the end of the lifespan of a photon, a million years, plus eight minutes, plus one second—to bring us the enjoyment of seeing the full moon. So, while I appreciate the sight of the full moon, I also think about the millions of photons ending their existence in my retina to supply me this enjoyable illumination. Out on the ocean, my scientific understanding enhanced the beauty all around me.

In my real-world daily activities, sometimes I get stuck in the science of what was happening in front of me. For example, once when I was taking a shower and observed the shower curtain moving inwards, I wondered if it was due to the wind from the open window or to the temporary vacuum created by the spraying water coming from the shower. I got out of the shower, closed the window, then got back into the shower to observe again. It was the vacuum.

I always try to fill the tank of my car early in the morning. It's cooler then, and cooler temperatures cause a slight increase of the density of gasoline. So, with gas measured by volume, I get slightly more gasoline in the cool early morning. The temperature difference in the underground depot is less than that at the surface. So, I don't save much, perhaps a nickel or dime. But I still fill up my car in the mornings.

When I'm making Turkish coffee, I listen to the sound of heating water resulting from the stress water endures with rising heat as water molecules speed up. Once it starts boiling however, the stress and the sound vanish, and the temperature stays the same (100 degrees Celsius or 212 degrees Fahrenheit at sea level). I know that gives me about ten seconds to remove the coffee pot from the stove before the coffee overflows. So I don't have to wait in front of the stove when brewing Turkish coffee; I go about my business while listening for the sound of the heating water.

When I add cream or sugar to coffee or tea, I stir the solution with a spoon. The sound made by the mixing spoon hitting the cup changes pitch as the density of the liquid increases. After a while, the sound stays the same. Then I know the solution is fully mixed, and I can stop stirring. Science helps me function efficiently, too!

* * *

When I returned from the cruise, slightly heavier despite avoiding alcohol, I had a message from the Santa Rosa Junior College (SRJC) inviting me for an interview. The interview went well. Even though my professional career was in industry with limited college teaching experience, they took a chance on me and extended an offer. I would teach general chemistry labs several times a week.

Meanwhile, Sibel completed her first three semesters at the Global Studies Program in Germany, South Africa, and India; and she found a not-for-profit company in San Francisco for her summer internship. That would make four continents that she lived in during a time span of one year. And I thought *I* was a global traveler!

She stayed with me for the summer and commuted to work on weekdays. This gave us an opportunity to have fun together on weekends. One weekend, we would walk around the streets of San Francisco following a map of all the interesting mural art on the walls of old buildings. Another weekend, we would visit the floating homes of Sausalito and take a sailing tour of the Bay. We also hung out around Burlingame, and she joined me hiking several of my favorite scenic trails.

The creativity Sibel exhibited as a kid hadn't faded. During her first semester in Freiburg, she was staying at a dormitory in a unit with six students and decided to paint a mural on the walls of the shared living room. It was a corner piece, a flowering spring tree on the left, and bare branches on the right, with leaves flying away from these branches. The name of each roommate was inscribed on the leaves flying off.

At the end of the summer of 2016, she returned to Freiburg to write her thesis and finish her master's program. When she returned to Freiburg and visited her old dorm, she discovered that the students who had lived there after her had drawn additional flying leaves on the wall with their names inscribed. Without realizing it, Sibel had started a new tradition.

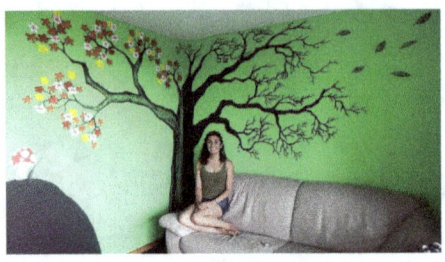

Sibel posing in front of the mural she created; the flying leaves represent the resident students moving out

Sibel finished her master's degree in Freiburg with a relatively small graduating class. Though I couldn't make the trip to Freiburg, I watched the graduation online since Sibel delivered the commencement speech. After graduation, she wanted to travel around Europe while applying for jobs there, though that didn't work out. She received a job offer from the company where she had done her internship in San Francisco and returned to the Bay Area.

\* \* \*

I was assigned two labs to teach for my first semester in Santa Rosa. Then, due to a last-minute cancellation, they needed an instructor and asked if I could do a third lab session at the Petaluma campus of SRJC. I said yes. So, I leased an apartment in Rohnert Park about midway between Santa Rosa and Petaluma. The semester started two weeks before I moved there, so I had a hellish two weeks with a two-hour commute each way.

When I moved, Sibel was towards the end of her internship and still with me, and Kurt also came over to help me move. We leased a U-Haul truck, packed everything into it, cleaned up the old apartment, and moved to Rohnert Park, about 45 miles north of San Francisco. The new place had a large patio, so I purchased some patio furniture before we returned the U-Haul truck. It was nice to have Kurt and Sibel together, and when our work was done, we scoped out some of the restaurants in Rohnert Park. Kurt returned to Salt Lake City the next day, and Sibel to Freiburg a week later.

# CHAPTER 13

# At Santa Rosa Junior College

*Santa Rosa, California, 2016-2021*

Before I started putting together my lectures, I wanted to make sure that I followed the college's standards. I asked around about a template for PowerPoint presentations with the university logo and branding. Nobody seemed to understand what I was asking for. Didn't they have a unified template for presentations by the university personnel? In industry, companies typically use consistent templates to keep their brand strong. Was that not the case at SRJC? Eventually, a faculty member explained to me that, due to concerns for academic freedom, everybody did their own thing. So I developed my own template with the university logo on top and a bar underneath in university colors. Voila! I had my standard template. Now I could put together my lectures.

During my first semester, a college-wide email solicited titles for presentations for the next semester's Professional Development Activities Day (PDA). I was excited to be at SRJC and so decided to contribute to the PDA. I proposed two titles: "Leadership vs. Management: Understanding the Difference may Help with Your Career Advancement" and "Treating the Disease, not just the Symptoms."

I could put together the first presentation using some of my material from Accelrys where I had given workshops for my product managers.

The second one would tap into some of my recent research at Mercer University. The PDA organizers accepted the first one but not the second because it didn't address professional development. Though I saw their point, I didn't fully agree because the topic is important for anyone dealing with health problems, which can certainly affect your professional development. I was disappointed but accepted their decision.

At the PDA, I delivered my leadership vs. management presentation to an audience of only sixteen people, with few questions at the end. Based on feedback I received, I realized that the audience had not understood my main points. It seemed I had failed to connect with my audience; I had forgotten my own insight about needing to change focus midstream if I perceived that I was losing my audience. I found the whole experience disappointing.

I attended some of the other PDA sessions. One that was of particular interest to me was about undergraduate research programs. It was a good session describing some of the biology department's activities; I suggested that computational chemistry could lend itself to many interesting research projects for undergraduate level chemistry students. We could streamline such an initiative at a low cost for some hardware, software, and a room for a computational chemistry lab. The participants seemed excited about these ideas during the PDA meeting, but nothing came of it. None of the tenured faculty seemed interested in sponsoring my suggestions, and I held little sway as only a part-time instructor.

Later in the semester, I heard that the Oakwood Sunday Lecture Series was looking for speakers. For this community of mostly retired people, lectures every Sunday featured speakers ranging from politicians to local celebrities to scientists. Speakers received a small honorarium. I sent the title that had been rejected by the PDA, "Treating the Disease, not just the Symptoms," and it was accepted by the Oakwood organizers.

The lecture hall was large, and the audio/visual equipment was modern. I presented to an audience of about a hundred people. The relatively long question-and-answer session included some intriguing discussions. Some of the questions revealed a highly informed audience. It was a good day.

* * *

Having taken general chemistry some forty years ago, I had to relearn it so that I could teach it effectively. I enjoyed doing this. I discovered many intriguing aspects of chemistry that I had forgotten. I would spend nine to twelve hours on campus (labs, lectures, office hours), and an additional ten hours or so preparing classes at home. The twenty or so hours a week of fulfilling work paid enough to cover the rent on the apartment and the utilities, so I only had to pull a small amount from my retirement account to augment my income. I could continue to do this, at least, until I would be fully vested in my social security retirement in June 2022. At that point, six years' out, I would, I thought, retire in Turkey.

I typically requested to teach early morning classes. Students taking these classes usually needed to go to work after class and tended to be relatively mature. But I would also get the occasional high school student taking my class as an advanced placement class. In one class, a high school student ended up being my best student.

I had a gamut of personalities, from aggressive students who were demanding of my time with their questions and debates and who would struggle throughout the semester, to silent students who never ask any questions but would get top exam scores and deliver picture-perfect lab reports.

One semester an autistic student, Ian, sat right up front. He seemed well-adjusted to the class social setting. He would make eye contact when talking with me and was not shy asking questions in class (which to me seemed unusual for a kid with autism). He had an occasional stutter. All the students were patient and waited until he completed his questions. He was curious and involved with the class.

Ian showed me his notebook once. I think he wanted to practice setting up a dimensional analysis (aka unit analysis) of mathematical equations given a set of conditions (e.g., given such and such a reaction, how many grams of carbon dioxide are released if you burn ten grams of sugar). He had completed the calculation for one set up, then repeated the same calculation for another, then another. With tiny writing, he repeated the same calculation for slightly different conditions perhaps over a hundred times. It was amazing. He must have spent hours doing that. Perhaps this was his process for learning.

He once came to my office riding a unicycle. A unicycle? Ian never stopped surprising me. In one of the exams, he was running out of time to complete the exam. However, I had an accommodation letter that allowed me to give him additional time for the exam. Since another class was coming into the room, I took him to the shared office for the adjunct faculty and had him complete the exam there. When he gave me the answer sheet, I noticed that he had not filled out the last six questions. This was a multiple-choice exam. I suggested that he not leave any of the questions unanswered and to just randomly select an answer for those unfilled questions, so he'd have a reasonable chance of getting one or two right. He complied.

Ian had to miss a couple of classes to join his father who gave seminars about autism. His father, Hank Smith, had authored a book entitled "Sticks and Stones, A Father's Journey into Autism." I purchased the book and read it. It was about his experiences raising Ian. After the final exam, I asked Ian to sign it for me. He did. Then he asked if I wanted him to also draw a flower or something next to his signature. I said he did not need to draw a picture (though later, I wished I had said yes). He finished the semester with a B grade. This autistic student was well on his way to becoming a productive and successful member of society. I was proud of Ian. I still remember him with fondness.

I like students who are interactive. Especially since I still teach, but now, online classes. In those I virtually pose a problem and give time for students to evaluate it. They respond, commenting and reacting through a chat window. Their feedback helps me with the pacing, so that I can slow down or speed up depending on how quickly I see the students are following along. Because all of my online classes are video recorded, when students do miss something, they can always go back to the recording and watch the presentation at their own pace.

* * *

Even though I didn't do any research after I left Atlanta, my colleagues there and I continued to publish papers about the research that I had performed there. For the next four to five years after my departure, I coauthored a couple of papers per year. The delay in publishing was because my research was on the front end of multi-disciplinary, multi-university, multi-year projects. The biologically active new chemical entities we found at the Center for Drug Design would first be biologically assessed at a collaborating university before a group from yet another university synthesized analogs of the lead compounds. The researchers who initially assessed the new compounds would now assess these analogs, and so on. By the time we were ready to publish, some three to five years would have passed since I finished my part. So I kept publishing, years after I stopped researching.

In one of these papers, a coauthor was an undergraduate student from one of the community colleges in Atlanta. I thought, "why couldn't that undergraduate student be from SRJC?" If I could set up a computational chemistry lab as I had discussed at the PDA, we could involve students in these research projects. To train the students, we could offer a new course entitled "Introduction to Molecular Modeling." The following semester, we could teach the students about research and have them work with professors at SRJC on some of their ongoing research projects. These would be short, one-semester undergraduate projects. This way they could earn co-authorships in peer-reviewed scientific papers even before they left SRJC. Imagine the marketing value to SRJC of being able to transfer students to four-year colleges as published authors or patented inventors, not to mention the value to the students themselves.

I was convinced that the undergraduate research concept I had proposed at the PDA was feasible. It would require a lot of work: founding the computational chemistry lab, creating the new "Molecular Modeling" course, establishing several long-term research projects with my former collaborators. But first I would need to convince SRJC leadership to fund and support the initiative. However, I couldn't do it as a part-time employee with limited time on campus.

* * *

Every summer, I would go to Turkey and try to stay there for at least a month. I could afford long visits since I didn't teach summer semesters. Kurt and Emily would visit every third year or so. During one of their visits, we took a road trip together, four of us: Emily, Kurt, my mom, and me. We started from Marmaris and headed north. Our first stop was the resort town of Kuşadası, where we enjoyed the sights along the Aegean Sea. The next morning, we drove to Ephesus, a UNESCO World Heritage Site and one of the world's best-preserved ancient cities. One can easily spend a full day touring inside the city walls. When we were there, workers were excavating a newly discovered part called Terraces, where wealthy people had lived. We paid the extra fee to get in. The residences arrayed along an incline, each row of homes slightly higher than the previous row. Ancient mosaics decorated the floors, slowing the excavation and cleanup process. I made a mental note to come back again to see the exhibit in all its colorful splendor once the work was completed. The large amphitheater at Ephesus, with room for 25,000 people and incredible acoustics, was well maintained. You can hear a whisper from the stage all the way at the back of the amphitheater.

Kuşadası is a popular stop for cruise ships, and the tour of Ephesus is one of the most popular excursions, though these tours are often so rushed that visitors don't even know what they're missing.

Two other sites in the area are worth exploring: The Temple of Artemis, one of the Ancient Seven Wonders of the World, though only one column of the temple still stands, and the House of the Virgin Mary, considered the last home of Mary, mother of Jesus. Of the two, we only had time to visit Mary's house.

Next, we headed further north to Pergamon. Here, half a dozen widely spread sites make it wise to allow ample time to visit. If you allocate a half day for each, you'll need three days to see all the major sites. We had only one day so limited our visits to one ancient site,

Asklepion, and one museum, the Pergamon Museum. Asklepion was an important health treatment center in antiquity. The site contains remains of a theater, courtyard, library, and temple. There would have also been sleeping rooms, sacred spring baths, and a long underground tunnel to protect the wealthy clients from the climate when they walked from place to place. Terraces in Ephesus and Asklepion in Pergamon together make vivid the privileged lifestyle of the rich and powerful of ancient times.

Our last stop was Bodrum, the site of the Mausoleum at Halicarnassus, another one of the Seven Wonders of the Ancient World. Emily wanted to visit the Bodrum Museum of Underwater Archeology. Unfortunately, it was closed for restoration. Hülya and Kemal had a house just outside Bodrum that provided an excellent closure to a great road trip.

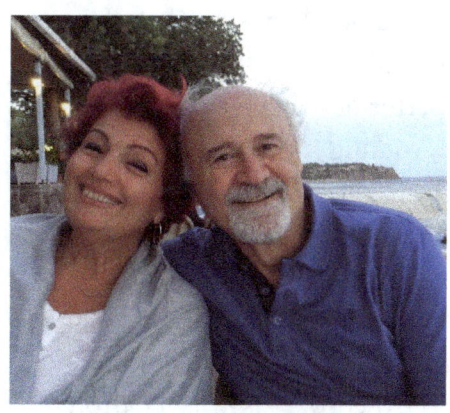

**Hülya and Kemal**

Hülya had prepared a feast suitable for Ottoman Sultans, over which we reminisced about our college adventures. Kurt and Emily got to meet my best friends of some forty years and heard stories I had long forgotten. Late that night, we drove the last three hours back to Marmaris.

* * *

Back in California, life went on at SRJC, with an addition to my general chemistry responsibilities. After a last-minute cancellation, on short notice the chemistry department was desperately looking for someone to teach one of the organic chemistry lab sections. I agreed to do it for two semesters. My academic training in organic chemistry made refreshing my memory on the fundamentals enjoyable.

Unlike the general chemistry students with one lab session per week, organic chemistry students had two lab sessions as most experiments would take the two sessions to complete. They also had to conduct spectroscopic analyses of their newly synthesized compounds so would have to spend extra time after the lab running the instruments (we could never complete the spectroscopic analyses within the time allotted for the labs). Fourier-transform Infra-Red spectroscopy (FTIR), Nuclear Magnetic Resonance spectroscopy (NMR), and Gas chromatography-Mass spectrometry (GCMS) were those advanced tools the students used most frequently to analyze the compounds they had synthesized. Organic chemistry was the highest-level chemistry course at SRJC, which meant that the students were afterwards ready to move on from community college to four-year programs. I wrote several recommendation letters for students transferring to university or applying for summer internships. Several years later, I wrote a few more recommendation letters for some of them who were moving on to graduate programs. I like to think I may have helped inspire some of those choices.

In the second semester of that organic chemistry class, I set up a friendly competition between the students. At the end of each experiment, I would name the top performer of that experiment and bestow on that person (or a pair if working in partnership) an award with a funny made-up name. For example, for the experiment involving a Friedel Crafts reaction, the winner earned the title "Crafty-Friedel," while for the experiment involving the Suzuki reaction, the winner earned the title "Suzuki-the-MAN." Similarly, some of the other made-up titles were: "Master of Borohydride," "Do I Brominate or What?" "Benzoin Maker," "I know my Spectroscopy," "Nitrile Hydrolyzer," and "Natural Acid Synthesizer." At the end of the semester, the person who had collected the most points would also earn the title "Green-Thumbs-of-Organic-Synthesis."

In the final project of the semester, the students practiced authoring a scientific paper. They adopted a "pet molecule" and drafted a short article about it, its significance and synthesis details with a full bibliography in the American Chemical Society (ACS) format for publishing papers in scientific journals. In the last part of this project, the students gave a short oral presentation on their Pet Molecule. I organized a symposium, like the scientific symposia that I used to organize when I was involved in the ACS technical program. Before they delivered their oral presentations, for each speaker, I provided a brief introduction that included all the funny titles they had earned during the lab sessions. The students loved it. They took the project seriously. Some even dressed professionally to deliver their presentations.

About a year later, a couple of my former organic students brought me a gift. It was a bottle of wine whose real label showed the organic chemistry of wine making. I was thrilled and saved the bottle. Years later, when I left Santa Rosa and drove to Salt Lake City to visit Kurt, that bottle of wine was in my car. After spending two days in the hot car, I doubt that the wine survived. So, I never actually tasted the wine. Another year later when I was visiting Kurt and Emily, they gave me a framed copy of the wine label as a gift. They had requested it from the winery that made the wine and then framed for me.

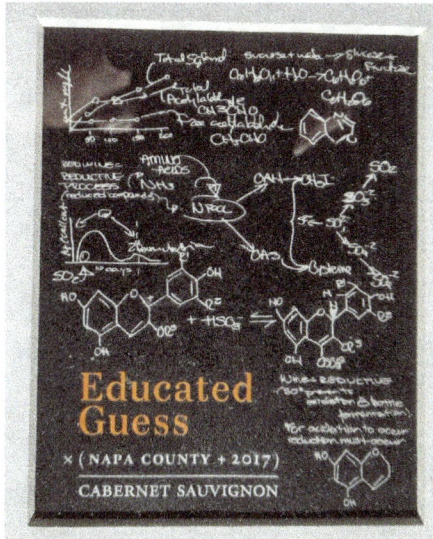

The label of the wine bottle showing the organic chemistry of wine; My organic chemistry students gave me a bottle of this wine, and my kids later gave me this framed label

After the first two semesters in SRJC, all my classes were at the Santa Rosa campus. To reduce my commute time, I moved there and rented an apartment just twelve minutes away from the campus. I settled into a routine and enjoyed the natural beauty of Northern California.

\* \* \*

When I left for Turkey for the first time in 2010, I had given my convertible to Kurt. Now he remembered how much I had enjoyed driving it around California and offered it back. He wasn't driving it in the cold, harsh climate of Salt Lake City. It was collecting dust in his carport. So I drove the car back to California following my next visit. Sibel joined me, and we had a pleasant road trip back with an overnight stay around Lake Tahoe. I hiked most Wednesdays, and these excursions became more fun when I drove with the top down through the amazing redwood forests and beautiful scenery of Northern California. I enjoyed the car until I finally left Santa Rosa, selling it a few days before my final departure to Turkey, 16 years after I bought it.

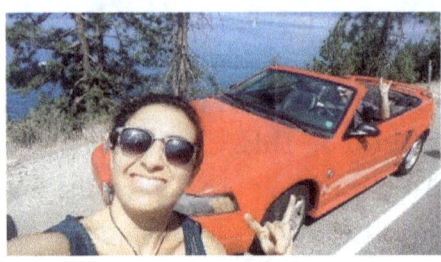

**At Lake Tahoe, during our road trip back to California, with Sibel**

While in Santa Rosa, I gave ballroom dancing another shot. I took an intermediate dance class nearby and also signed up for a beginners' salsa class a short drive away in Petaluma. Even though I was still struggling, learning two vastly distinctive styles of dance worked out well for me. I was not as stiff as before and started taking more chances with the moves and escaping routine.

The final class I took was a more advanced, fast-moving class. The instructor focused on developing a choreographed routine that involved up to a dozen different moves. Every three to four weeks, we learned choreographed moves for a different dance, including waltz, rumba, cha-cha, tango, salsa, foxtrot, swing, and probably a few more that I can't remember. Once I realized that a sequence of moves from one dance could be adapted to another, I would try them out and enjoy the outcome when it worked.

Another attractive aspect of this last class was my classmates. After each class, we would all go to a restaurant in the area and hang out. I not only learned about all the good restaurants in the area, but also socialized with a group, which was out of character for me. One couple from the group, Allan and Marilyn, were exceptionally good dancers and good people. Allan was blind, but this didn't hinder his dancing. The instructor would accommodate him when teaching the moves, and this little bit extra was enough for him to adapt and learn with the rest of us.

When Allan and Marilyn joined a conversation, the intellectual quality climbed a notch. I remember one story Marilyn told about dancing at a salsa club. They were caught up in the music, thoroughly enjoying the dancing, and having a lot of fun with it. At the end of the music, when they stopped, everybody was clapping and cheering for them. At a certain point, all the other couples on the dance floor noticed the joy radiating from Marilyn and Allan and formed a circle around them to watch. I guess that not many of them even knew that Allan was blind.

* * *

Once a week, on Wednesdays, I would go hiking, exploring the many different trails around Santa Rosa. One of my favorite places was Bodega Bay, the site of Hitchcock's famous movie *The Birds*. I would hike the Bodega Head trails (see the front cover picture) and often have my lunch at the Spud Point Crab Company. They cook the best clam chowder, but my favorite was their crab cocktail. I would order takeout, park my Mustang at a scenic waterfront spot and enjoy my lunch.

My second favorite Wednesday excursion was to Jenner, a small coastal town of little more than 100 people. I'd have my coffee and breakfast at the Café Aquatica where I enjoyed the beautiful scenery of the Russian River reaching the Pacific Ocean. Then, I would hike either in the Jenner Mountains or drive the scenic Route-1 South to Bodega Bay. The route from Jenner to Bodega Bay, offered about a dozen different scenic trails to choose from.

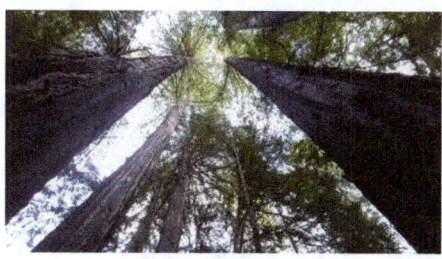
Redwoods... my favorite trees

I also found several routes near home to walk for exercise. The apartment complex was well designed with over a hundred redwood trees spread throughout the complex. Returning from my walks, I would enter the complex from the back and walk through some of the older and larger redwood trees. Around one corner, I could reach the lower branches of a smaller but proud-looking redwood tree.

I would gently caress its needle-like leaves and whisper terms of endearment. I pretended that it could hear me and appreciated the kindness. Such was my year-long relationship with "George," the redwood tree.

On Bodega Head sits a large, distinct cypress tree that dwarfs its neighbors and is visible from any location on that promontory into the Pacific. One day, as I passed by the tree, I noticed a hawk perched on one of its hidden branches. From that point on, I routinely stopped there; I would find "George," the hawk and, when no one was around, gently talk to him. We would make eye contact briefly, but he would quickly look away, perhaps glimpsing his next potential meal. Our affection seemed to be one directional. George wouldn't indulge me. He would ignore me mostly. But probably because he knew that he could fly away any time, he tolerated me coming close to take photos or to talk. After several months, I felt we had developed a friendship of sorts.

One day, when I arrived at Bodega Head, I was horrified at the sight of the large cypress tree blown down by an intense storm the previous day. The large branches of the tree were scattered around on the ground, with only a bare trunk left, and George was nowhere to be found. I was devastated. The next week, George was still missing, but he showed up the following week standing on the highest point of the stub and looking down on people. Unfortunately, since he was now unhidden, he was quickly discovered by visitors to the area. They came to the remains of the cypress tree to take photos and shoot selfies. This attention bothered George and he left, this time for good.

Three weeks later, I found him about five miles north of Bodega Bay during a coastal trail hike there. I think it was George since he let me approach to take a photograph, which matched my earlier photos. This was the last time I saw George. But I was happy that he was moving in the right direction. Another eight miles north, and he would make it to the Jenner Mountains and the sizable community of hawks there. He would be right at home with his fellow raptors.

Later, during my last weeks in Santa Rosa, Sibel stayed with me and helped with the stuff that I needed to get rid of before my final move to Turkey. On one of my Wednesday excursions, she went with me to Jenner, where we had coffee and snacks at Café Aquatica. Then we headed north to the Jenner Mountains. Two trails, "Sea to Sky," and "Raptor Valley," make a nice loop just over five miles long. The highest point opened to a hundred-and-eighty-degree vista of the scenery below. On one of my earlier hikes, I had met a group of people at that vista point, members of a nature club who were recording and watching the hawk population. Several hawks flew in groups of three or four.

I was hoping to catch such a scene, so recommended to Sibel that we hike the loop. When we reached the vista point on top, we spent some time looking for hawks in the hope of spotting George among them. I wanted Sibel to meet my friend George, however we didn't see any hawks. Disappointed, we continued the hike, and had to pass through a herd of large Angus cattle. We also sighted a mountain lion from a distance; Sibel was able to record a video of it. Further down into the valley, we finally sighted a group of three hawks flying around. We hoped that one of them was George, but none of them approached us, so we weren't sure.

* * *

My grandson, Ziya, was born on November 17, 2019. I was a grandfather! He was small in size and weight, but healthy, and he has since met all of his physical milestones. Ziya gave me the chance to see Kurt as a father. He was all in, from changing diapers, to washing and clothing Ziya. I had also performed such tasks occasionally when Kurt was a baby. But not as much, with Zeynep as the homemaker at that time, and me working long hours at work. My working hard to make ends meet and pay for our lifestyle forced the separation of roles in our nuclear family. Over the years, I ended up regretting the time that I spent away from my children as they grew. Now I was glad for Kurt, whose empathetic and gentle personality helped him find and develop his parenting skills naturally.

Shortly after he became a father, Kurt graduated with his PhD in history. Following his final oral defense, his dissertation committee met Ziya, who was waiting just outside the door in the arms of his mom.

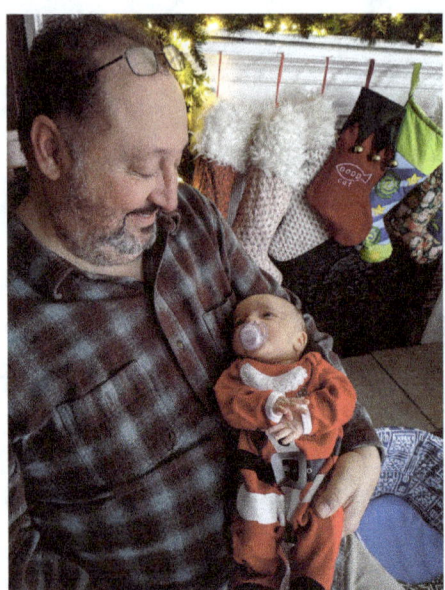

My first holidays with Ziya (when he was two months old)

\* \* \*

Towards the middle of the spring 2020 semester, a viral infection started to spread around the world, causing what would come to be called Covid-19. This was worrisome, and the SRJC administration had to decide, during the spring break, how to continue the classes. But then Covid-19 was declared a worldwide pandemic and the university administration decided to close all campuses. We would have to finish classes online. Most of us received a crash-course in online teaching, and we came through. By the time the semester was over, the Covid-19 pandemic reached serious levels in the US with businesses closing and industries like hospitality and restaurants in shutdown. The summer semester was canceled while the administration tried to figure out how to continue educating our students in the future. Most classes would be taught online, but the labs were a different story. Their hands-on aspect was an important part of the chemical education, so the university settled on a hybrid process where one-third of the lab sessions would be in-person.

The school implemented strict safety protocols for these in-person lab sessions. The students and faculty alike would go through a safety check before they were allowed to enter the lab. Everyone was in full compliance, and the in-person lab sessions during the first semester of pandemic teaching ended with no recorded Covid-19 cases. We were able to adjust to the new conditions and managed to continue the education, despite the limitations forced upon us by the pandemic.

The situation at home was a bit less fun for me since I lived alone. After a year, the social isolation was getting stale. Being away from my family both in Utah and in Turkey during such trying times made things difficult. At least Sibel was relatively close by in Berkeley, but we couldn't meet during the lockdowns. We kept in close contact with each other, via Skype, Zoom, and WhatsApp, and all of us got our Covid-19 vaccinations as soon as we were eligible. Except for groceries (most of which would be delivered, but occasionally, I would make the trip to shop), I would not leave home at all and delivered all my online classes from my home office. My only outings were my Wednesday excursions. These kept me sane during a period of depressive social isolation.

The situation in Turkey was also dire, if not worse. My mom reached the age of ninety and was dealing with a multitude of health problems in addition to the social isolation. She had a heart-rhythm disorder called tachycardia. After trying several different drugs, her doctor had settled on Isoptin®, which seemed to work, though it took her some months to acclimate to it. Every now and then, she would have a fleeting episode of an exceedingly high heartrate, and the doctor had to keep adjusting the dosage to find the best treatment regimen. Eventually her condition stabilized. The drug she was using, however, was an old drug no longer manufactured in Turkey. Mine ended up systematically calling all the pharmacies in Ankara and buying the medicine from those who happened to have it in stock. Mom and Mine lived in the same apartment building one floor apart. So having my sister close to Mom helped them to get through the lockdowns. Beyond helping Mom with groceries and doctor visits, she would visit her every afternoon to play card games and gossip. I was grateful that Mine was able to hold down the fort during this dangerous pandemic. Being away from Mom during this crisis was the last straw for me. I decided to scrap my original plan and accelerate my relocation back to Turkey instead of waiting for my Social Security checks to start.

Once I decided to move soon, implementing my new plan was straightforward. I donated everything in my household to charities. I attempted to resign from SRJC, vacated the apartment in Santa Rosa, drove to Salt Lake City to visit Kurt and his family, and finally took a one-way flight to Turkey. Sibel stayed with me during my last two weeks in Santa Rosa and was a tremendous help with my relocation.

During the pandemic, my dance sessions had of course been canceled. Following a year's isolation, our group came together for the first time, for a last luncheon to send me off to Turkey. The photograph is from this lunch meeting.

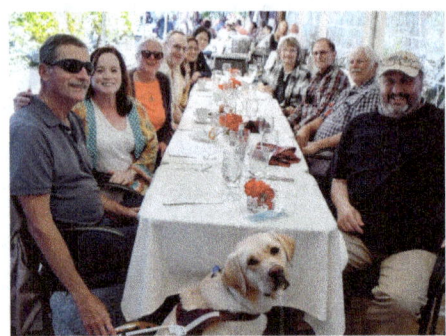

The dance group: Alan and Marilyn sitting front left; I'm at front right. Sibel took the photo.

The chemistry department chair at SRJC suggested that rather than resign I simply take a leave of absence. That way we would have time to see how things developed. If I eventually did decide to come back, I could continue to work for SRJC and avoid the whole job application process. I was pleased at his attempts to keep me engaged. I felt flattered. He later revised his recommendation slightly and suggested that, instead of taking a leave of absence, I should simply request to teach only online classes with a simulated lab component.

Considering that Turkey has stable internet access, I thought this plan might work. I requested to teach a general chemistry online class where my lectures would be 7:30 - 9:00 a.m. Tuesdays and Thursdays, and the simulated lab sessions would be at 9:00 a.m. - noon on Tuesdays. The time difference was not much of a problem for early morning classes since Turkey was ten hours ahead of California. So 7:30 a.m. in California was 5:30 p.m. in Turkey, a good time for me.

After three years in Berkeley, Sibel was getting restless. As an adult, she hadn't lived in one place for longer than a year before now. She decided to get another master's degree, this time in environmental science. She selected the University of Cape Town in South Africa, where she had studied for one semester during her first master's and enjoyed the decolonial approach to education, as well as the relatively low tuition fees. Because of the pandemic, the campus was closed, so she completed the first semester online while still at Berkeley. I tried to persuade her to do a PhD instead, but she didn't think she could stay in one place for four years. I guess three years is her location limit.

* * *

I was assuming that my new move to Turkey would be permanent. However, my last move eleven years earlier was intended to be permanent too, yet I had returned to the US in two years. After the disruptions of Covid-19, it seemed anything could happen. My children and their families were in the US, while my mom, Mine and their families were in Turkey. Perhaps a hybrid solution, say living six months at each location, was a possibility.

I was heading to Turkey to start the next chapter of my life after 50, another life milestone. I had first come to the US in 1982 and now I was returning to Turkey thirty-nine years later in 2021.

# CHAPTER 14

# Back to Turkey

*Marmaris, Turkey, 2021-present*

In June 2021, I flew back to Turkey. I stayed in Ankara for a week to run some errands and get myself set up. The errands included getting a new cell phone, setting up my bank account with the new phone number so that I could continue with online banking, getting some personal electronics (beard trimmer, toothbrush, etc.) with the right power plugs, and getting new tires for Mom's car. Then I drove that car to Marmaris, where Mom and I intended to spend the rest of the year together. Mom, Mine, and her husband were already there for the summer. A little later, my sister's son and his family with their new puppy visited. They stayed in the hotel next door but were often with us. They wanted to spend time with Mom, Grandma, and their uncle. Suddenly, I was amongst chaos and social activity. You can perhaps appreciate the magnitude of this change for me, someone who had lived alone for the past fifteen years.

Meanwhile, Sibel made it to Cape Town, and, after a short acclimation period, she started her second semester there. Her boss in the US not only allowed her to work online for another three months while in Cape Town, but the kind woman also rolled the cost of the US benefits she was no longer using into her salary for this period, essentially giving her a raise. Bosses like her do still exist, though it seems they're an endangered species. Sibel had to deal with the rise of the Omicron variant of Covid-19 in Cape Town. Somehow, my family have all survived the pandemic so far without catching it. Sibel had her second southern hemisphere summer-New Year's Eve in Cape Town. She is aiming to finish her thesis by the end of the fall of 2022.

* * *

Even though I usually preferred to be alone, when I was, I never felt lonely. Conversely, sometimes I would feel lonely when I was in the center of a crowd. During my time at Atlanta, I had looked forward to the university experience after some fifteen years working in industry. Perhaps, I thought back then, I would be more outgoing and develop some friendships. But even though I was interacting with people on the university campus, at the bridge club, and at backgammon tournaments, I discovered that I really didn't want to establish more intimate friendships; that was too much work. I was content being alone. This was something new I discovered about myself during that time, that I was not alone due to circumstance but rather by choice.

When I was playing bridge, I could be very sociable. When I was teaching on the cruise ships, I would interact with people readily and in the restaurants would chat with the wait staff. Sometimes even when I was out walking, I would interact with random people passing by in such a way that no one would think I prefer to be alone, but I do.

* * *

Before the start of the semester at Santa Rosa Junior College (SRJC) that I would teach from Turkey, I needed to set up a second phone line and internet connection in Marmaris, dedicated to my teaching activities. I needed a reliable and fast internet connection to hold my scheduled online classes. Mom was doing much better than I expected. The heart rhythm disorder stabilized. She had a mild fast-heartbeat episode only twice during the six months we were in Marmaris. However, within ten days of my arrival, she fell twice. Luckily, apart from a shoulder bruise, she was okay. Her other shoulder had a muscle tear from a fall a year earlier that the doctors could not treat since she was on a strong blood thinner. So she had learned to manage life even with the discomfort. Her repeated falling was a concern, especially since it had happened twice in one week. We persuaded Mom to use the nice cane a friend had given her as a gift whenever we went out. After a while, she stopped using her cane because she felt more stable on her own two feet. She has not fallen since then.

As Mom got on her feet, my classes at SRJC started and all was in order. The students were enthusiastic and actively took part in the class, responding to questions and participating in discussions. There had not been any technological connection problems. In the first class, I usually take time for the students to introduce themselves. I ask them to share their name, their major and what they want to do with it, their aspirations in life, and then one thing unique about themselves. During the in-person sessions, I would have the students pair up, interview each other, and introduce their partners to the class. For the on-line classes, I would simply have the individuals introduce themselves instead. In response to the question about their major, about a fourth reported that they were considering environmental science. At a time when we were dealing with rampant climate-change denial in the US, this interest by our young college students in environmental science was encouraging. Perhaps hope is alive for future generations.

I set up a Marmaris routine. Mornings I would go out for a walk on the boardwalk for about thirty minutes, then swim for about same amount of time, then have breakfast. Then I would start my workday at around 9:00 - 9:30 a.m. I would work several hours each day preparing for my classes throughout the week and then deliver the classes Tuesday and Thursday evenings. One of my reasons to return to Turkey early was to spend some quality time with Mom, and so we scheduled Friday evenings as date nights. We would go out for a dinner to one of the touristy restaurants on the boardwalk. We would eat gourmet food. Half the time that meant seafood. Mom loved fresh fish.

I was also able to catch up with some of my friends from our teenage days in Marmaris. Having moved into the condo fifty years earlier to spend our summers there, I had several friends from those days, some still around.

Selçuk and his family were our next-door neighbors. He was about my age, and we had hung out together during our summers in Marmaris. He was into electronics, and I was interested in that as well. At one period in my childhood, I was building radios and amplifiers from scratch. That was the extent of my involvement. Selçuk was much more deeply into it. One summer he came over with a radio transmitter that he had built. He said it was a small one with about a five-hundred-meter range (about a third of a mile). So, we set it up. I picked a cassette of popular music, and we started broadcasting. Then we grabbed a small portable transistor radio and started walking towards Marmaris listening to our broadcast. Our aim was to test the range of the transmission. At that time, radio broadcasting was illegal in Turkey. I was a freshman at Middle East Technical University (METU), and these were the times of political turmoil. We soon found ourselves in downtown Marmaris over a mile from home, and we were still broadcasting. Clearly the range of our broadcast was more than stated. Then we saw a police car rushing in the opposite direction. We panicked and thought that they were tracking our broadcast and were going to catch us. So, we hurried back home to stop the broadcast. On the way to our apartment, we noticed that one of the neighbors was listening to our music too. Finally, we made it home and stopped the broadcast. I wonder how many people listening had been disappointed when our music stopped.

This was some fifty years ago. So, when I heard that Selçuk was in town I contacted him, and we set up Wednesday nights as our dinner night. Whoever from our youth showed up, we would include them in our Wednesday dinner sessions, often reminiscing about the old days.

Sevtap and Hür were other familiar faces in town. They had had a house in the area but had sold it and bought one in Istanbul. However, they wanted to spend part of their summer in Marmaris and so leased an apartment in another complex for a month. Sevtap's family used to live in our complex and were our neighbors for many years. Hür was a friend from the METU chess club; he was one of the top players at METU. I had introduced them to each other, and they have been happily married for over forty years. We were all at or near retirement age, and our dinner conversations were mutually stimulating.

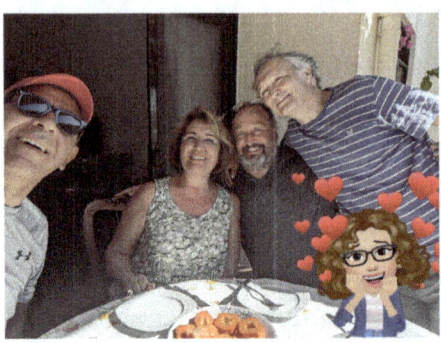

Selfie captured by Selçuk on the left, then Sevtap, me, and Hür

It was great to see old friends. We would dine in different restaurants every week, eventually settling on some favorites we returned to over and over. Our dinners would last four or five hours, and sometimes ended elsewhere for coffee or dessert. We would not order dinner all at once. First, we would order the starters and salads and work on them slowly for a while, then call the waiter over to order our main course which might be separate dishes for each, or shared courses, everyone serving themselves from the center of the table. We would typically consume a bottle or two of select wine. Then after the table was cleared (if we hadn't relocated) we would order dessert. Then we would have tea or coffee. By the time we were ready to pay the bill, we would be the last guests left in the restaurant. If this was a restaurant we'd been to before, the wait staff would know our process, and they would be very accommodating. Once, we had the chef visit our table to chat, and next thing we were served a fruit plate on the house. After Hür and Sevtap left, Selçuk and I continued with our Wednesday night dinners, afterwards sending our WhatsApp group a picture of our meeting. Then someone else we knew would show up in Marmaris, and they would be part of our Wednesday nights.

The day after the end of my semester at SRJC, Mom and I drove to Ankara. I had two days to get ready for my trip to Salt Lake City to join Kurt and family for the Christmas and New Year's holidays. Covid-19 protocols were in full effect. I had to show my vaccination card at the airport and also have a PCR test done within 24 hours of the start of my trip. I had had two shots of the Moderna vaccine, and I was due for my booster shot. Emily had already made an appointment for me for Monday morning the day after my arrival.

In Salt Lake City I found my grandson, Ziya, now two years old, was talking constantly. When I was making coffee in the kitchen, for example, he would announce to his parents in the living room that "Dede making coffee." Dede is Turkish for grandfather. My three weeks in Salt Lake City were amazing. My favorite times were in the evenings when I was putting Ziya down to bed. We would first read three or four of his favorite books, then have the Dede-Ziya dance while I whistled some lullaby tunes. He would keep looking at me while I was swaying in tune with my lullaby music, and gently play with my beard. Finally, Ziya would be in bed for his sleep.

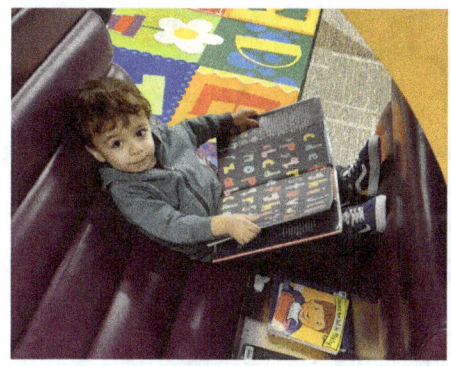
Two-year old Ziya in a local library

Kurt and Ziya would visit Zeynep on every other Sunday. Once she found out that I was in town, Zeynep invited me as well. With Emily also joining us, we had a family excursion. Zeynep had bought a house in Utah about an hour's drive from Kurt's. Ziya had a roomful of toys (some left over from his dad there. The lunch was great; I had forgotten how good a cook Zeynep is. I learned that she had been working for Northrop Grumman for the last twelve some years. This was our first time seeing each other since Kurt's wedding and it went well. I was happy to see her doing so well. My three weeks in Utah passed quickly, and I returned to Ankara.

* * *

I used my home office in Ankara for my classes. In the Spring semester, I had the same schedule for my lectures as I had for the fall semester: 7:30 – 9:00 a.m. (Pacific time). Being in Ankara, I was now able to join Mom and Mine for their afternoon card games.

Around this time, a distant uncle whom I didn't know well and who had been living in Istanbul, apparently in poverty in his late years, passed away. When some relatives looked at his bank accounts, they learned that Mine had been supporting him financially for the past two years. She had set up a bank account that would automatically transfer funds to his account every month. Mine hadn't mentioned what she was doing to anyone, and we wouldn't have found out about it if he hadn't passed away. This is who my sister Mine is. Despite being in a demanding marriage, she maintained a soft spot for people down on their luck.

* * *

Arriving in 1982 and leaving in 2021, I stayed in America for thirty-nine years (minus the two years I was in Turkey from 2010-12). I consider myself lucky to have witnessed and been professionally involved in the evolution of computer technology during that time. I served on an internet commission at Molecular Design Limited when browsers and public access to the internet were just starting. We wanted to evaluate commercial opportunities in case the internet became more popular. I was there when early personal computers became readily available. I was also there when supercomputers were on the rise. I was there for the start of cell phones, video conferencing, Siri, and satellite navigation. Like most of us back in the day, I knew how to read a map. Now how many of us can find an address today without the help of GPS?

The dramatic changes in how we apply technology, generation to generation, boggles the mind. If, when I first used computers, someone had said that I would be teaching a college course to a class seven-thousand miles away with audio and video, I wouldn't have believed it. I consider myself lucky for my remarkable journey through several paradigm-changing technological advancements.

* * *

During my stay in the US, I had made two critical career decisions with substantial consequences. The first one was around 1989 when I was finishing my postdoctoral fellowship in Alabama and resulted in me drastically changing my career path to go into industry—and marketing at that! And the second one was right after I started my consulting business in 2006. At that time, I had an opportunity to follow a natural progression of my career if I had taken the job offer from BioSolveIT. If I had done that, I would likely have remained in the corporate world for the next fifteen years and might even have broken the glass ceiling I had hit at Accelrys in another company. I would likely be retiring wealthy. *But would I have been happy?*

In my years in industry I had changed, a change catalyzed by Accelrys' unceremonious letting go of me. I realized that I wanted to do things that I liked to do, rather than the things that I was expected to do. So, in 2006, at that crossroad, I took a harder route, a more uncertain and riskier route. As a result, I retired with a modest income that will sustain only a modest lifestyle. But the same question applies. *Am I happy?*

\* \* \*

I hope in sharing my life after 50 I've inspired you to try to identify what is most important in life and, perhaps, start thinking about your end game. We all come to this world alone with nothing, and we will leave the same way. What we do in between deeply matters. Ultimately, our success will be measured not by the wealth we accumulate, but by our legacy, and how we will be remembered decades after our passing.

# Epilogue

**I am happy** knowing that my son, Kurt, is rooted in the US and has established his family there. He is already a far better father than I have been for my children.

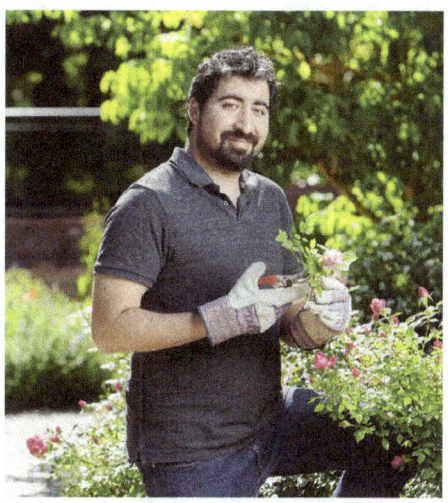

**Kurt gardening in Salt Lake City**

\* \* \*

**I am happy** knowing that my daughter, Sibel, will continue to travel around the world, not merely as a visitor but as someone who will integrate into the community at each stop and make a difference there.

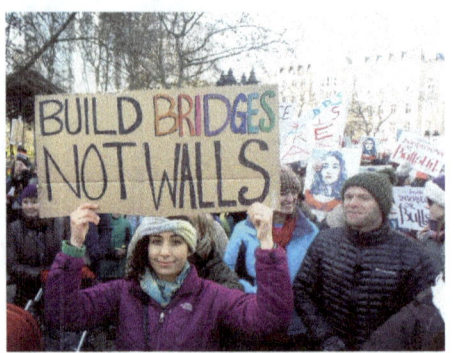

**Sibel at a rally in Frankfurt**

* * *

As for me, I remember my dream of thirty-three years ago, when my imagined granddaughter asked me what I had done with my life, and I was struggling with the answer of my career trajectory then: "I helped people develop better explosives." That dream forced me to re-evaluate my job options and resulted in me changing my scientific field and starting over. I still don't have a granddaughter, but at a future time when facing that question, I can now say, "I've helped people develop better medicines—and I've loved my life and the people in it."

**I am happy** knowing that I now have a much better answer.

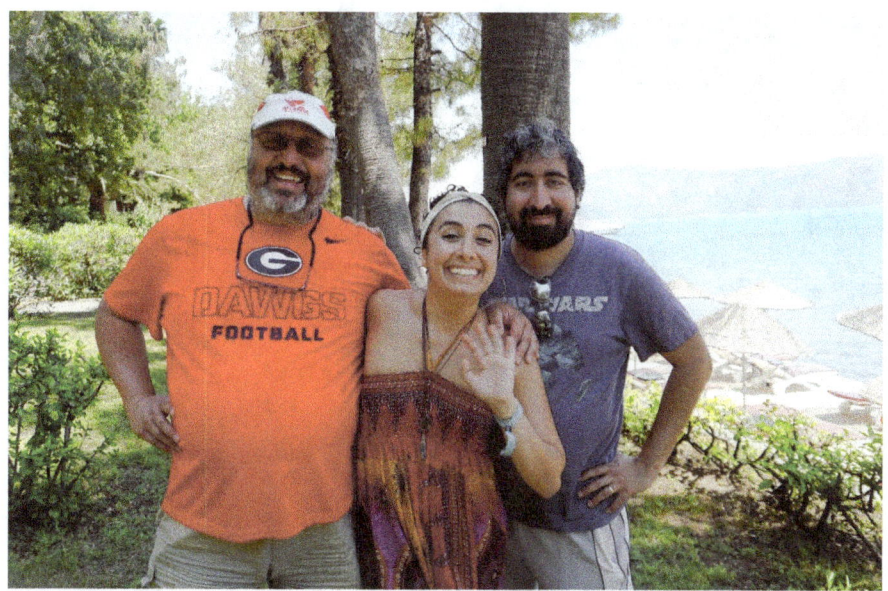

With Sibel and Kurt in Marmaris. The picture was taken by two-and-a-half-year-old Ziya playing with his aunt Sibel's camera. He liked the sound of the shatter when he pushed down a button.

The End

# APPENDIX I

## STEPWISE GENERATION OF THE PHARMACOPHORE MODEL FOR KMO INHIBITORS

When a three-dimensional (3D) structure of a target enzyme with a bound ligand is available, generating a pharmacophore model is simplified. The bound conformation supplies valuable information useful for generating the pharmacophore. Learn below about a stepwise approach for using this technology to discover new active compounds.

### Step 1: Identify a 3D structure of the target enzyme with a bound ligand.

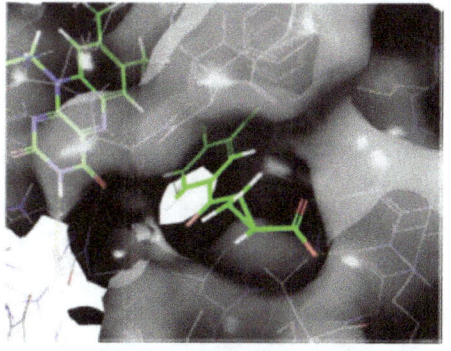

**The X-ray crystal structure complex of UPF 648 bound to yeast KMO.**
*Re-printed with permission from reference 33.*
*Copyright © 2017 Elsevier Inc.*

## Step 2: Extract the active ligand in its bound conformation.

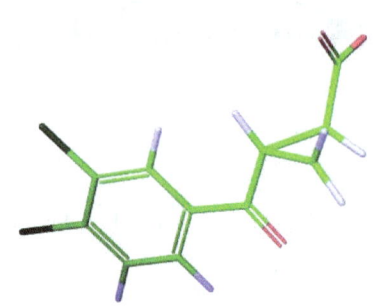

**UPF 648 extracted from the enzyme within its bound conformation**

## Step 3: Name and tag the features of the molecule that could interact with the receptor active site.

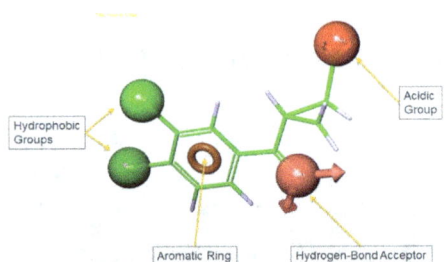

We identified five features as capable of potentially interacting with the KMO active site.

*Re-printed with permission from reference 34.*
*Copyright © 2022 MDPI*

## Step 4: Remove the ligand, while keeping the pharmacophoric features intact.

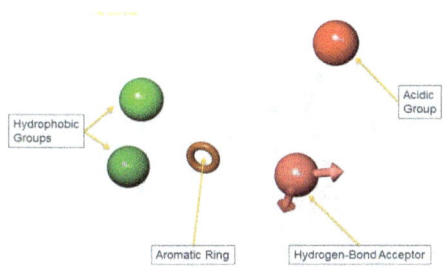

**Three-dimensional arrangement of the features of the UPF 648; i.e., This pharmacophore model was used to screen databases**

## Step 5: Search the 3D databases of commercially available chemicals to retrieve new potential KMO inhibitors.

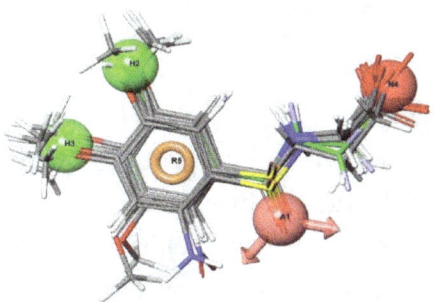

**Top 20 compounds retrieved from the Sigma/ Aldrich chemicals catalog.**
*Re-printed with permission from reference 34.*
*Copyright © 2022 MDPI*

## Step 6: *Prioritize the compounds in the hitlist for further consideration.*

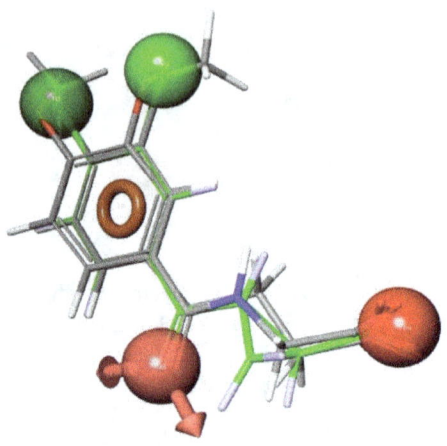

**The two lead compounds overlaid with UPF 648 (green). They both showed KMO inhibition at low micromolar levels.**
*Re-printed with permission from reference 33.*
*Copyright © 2017 Elsevier Inc.*

## Step 7 and beyond:

Optimize the lead compounds by generating synthetic novel analogs of them to increase the desired properties (e.g., potency) and decrease the undesired properties (e.g., toxicity). Our collaborators at the University of Georgia conducted the lead optimization.

PHARMACOPHORE MODEL GENERATION FOR NOX4
INHIBITORS AND NEW ACTIVE COMPOUNDS
RETRIEVAL

We followed several different lines of research; one strategy involved using some of the most active compounds identified in a published patent.

**Three compounds that inhibit Nox4 extracted
from patent literature**

Next we generated a pharmacophore model by flexibly aligning the three compounds and finding the common pharmacophoric features.

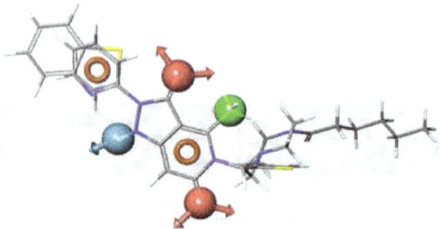

**The pharmacophore model had six features:
Two hydrogen-bond acceptors (pink), one
hydrogen-bond donor (blue), one lipophilic
group (green), and two aromatic ring
structures (orange).**
*Re-printed with permission from reference 35.
Copyright © 2017 Elsevier Inc.*

A search of commercially available chemicals databases with the pharmacophore model retrieved many compounds. However, most of those compounds had the same structural scaffold as the original compounds identified in the patent, which meant they were under patent protection.

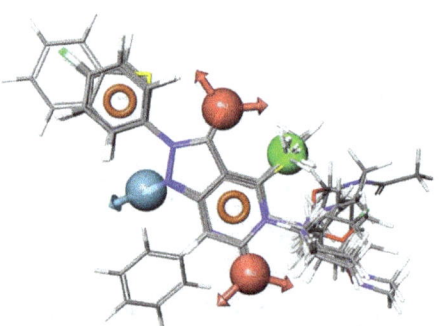

**Top 20 compounds retrieved with the
pharmacophore model, all under patent
protection by a competitor.**
*Re-printed with permission from reference 35.
Copyright © 2017 Elsevier Inc.*

However, two compounds further down on the hitlist fell outside patent protection, so we selected those two compounds for further study.

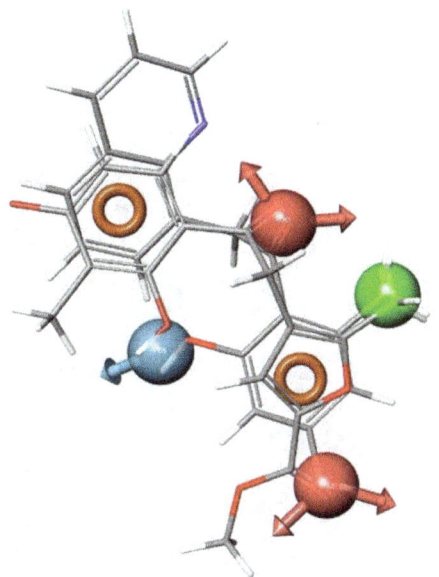

**The two lead compounds that were subjected
to lead optimization.**
*Re-printed with permission from reference 35.*
*Copyright © 2017 Elsevier Inc.*

## STEPWISE CREATION OF THE GÜNER-HENRY SCORE

Searching through a database of similar compounds infused with several active compounds is a good way to assess a pharmacophore model. Suppose you have a database of one-hundred compounds ($D = 100$) ten of which are known active compounds ($A = 10$). Then suppose you perform a search and retrieve twenty compounds ($Ht = 20$) with four active compounds in it ($Ha = 4$). Suppose you perform another search with a different model and retrieve thirty compounds ($Ht = 30$) with five active compounds ($Ha = 5$). Which hitlist is better? The one that retrieved four active compounds in a hitlist of twenty? Or the one that retrieved five active compounds in a hitlist of thirty?

We can evaluate the first search results that retrieved twenty hits, four of which are active, from a database of one hundred compounds. The sixteen compounds (i.e., $Ht - Ha = 16$) that matched the model but were not one of the known active compounds could be potentially active compounds that we did not know about. This is the promise of the approach. The best models are expected to yield a hitlist that may hold previously unknown active compounds.

Let us address the question of which model is better? The first or the second? Consider the ratio of active compounds to the hitlist, with percent yield as a metric: (%Y):

$$\%Y = \frac{Ha}{Ht} \times 100\%$$

You started with a database of one-hundred compounds, ten percent of which are known to be active (i.e., %Ydatabase= 10). Your first search retrieved twenty compounds with four actives (i.e., %Yfirst= 20). Hence, your hitlist is twice as enriched as the original database, with respect to active compounds. Your second search retrieved thirty compounds with five actives (i.e., %Ysecond= 16.7). Using percent yield as your metric, the first search is better with a score of 20 compared to the second search with 16.7. So if you use the first model to search a database of unknown compounds, the likelihood of retrieving an active compound with it is higher than with the second model.

One may take issue with this analysis since the second search retrieved five known active compounds while the first search retrieved only four. To address this, you could use another metric, say the percent of known active compounds retrieved: (%A):

$$\%A = \frac{Ha}{A} \times 100$$

Considering that the database has ten active compounds, the first search retrieved four active compounds (%Afirst= 40), while the second search retrieved five active compounds (%Asecond= 50). In this case, the second model seems better since it retrieved a higher percentage of active compounds. This conclusion is the opposite of the earlier analysis with %Y where the first model appeared better.

The conclusions differ depending on which metric one decides to use. This situation is unacceptable. Furthermore, both metrics fail in extreme cases. For example, if you get a hitlist containing one compound that you already knew was active, then %Y = 100. The first metric gives an astounding one-hundred percent score even though the result is useless (no potential new active compound). Another extreme case is a model that retrieves all the compounds in the database: then

%A =100. In this case the %A gives an astounding one-hundred percent score yet the hitlist is no better than the original database.

We needed a better metric. What if we combined these two metrics and called this new metric the Goodness of Hitlist Score, i.e., GH-Score (and later nicknamed the Güner-Henry score)? We easily obtained a linear combination of these two parameters by taking the average of these two metrics:

$$GH = \frac{\%Y + \%A}{2}$$

or

$$GH = \frac{\left(\frac{Ha}{Ht}\right) + \left(\frac{Ha}{A}\right)}{2}$$

This would be the case if both parameters, %Y and %A, were equal in importance. However, we found empirically that %Y is more important than %A by about three-fold. Hence:

$$GH = \frac{3 \times \left(\frac{Ha}{Ht}\right) + \left(\frac{Ha}{A}\right)}{2}$$

Working out the algebra, we get:

$$GH = \left(\frac{Ha \times (3A + Ht)}{4Ht \times A}\right)$$

This was the first form of the GH-Score. Doug Henry and I would attend the Gordon Research Conferences as roommates, either the one on computational chemistry or more likely the one on computer-aided drug design. Face time with Doug during these conferences helped me clarify my ideas floating around the GH-Score. At the end of one of these conferences, Doug and I set up the above rendition of the GH-Score.

In this form, it seemed to work well, though some questions remained about the quality of the results depending on whether they were obtained by searching an exceptionally large database or an exceedingly small one. We could make an adjustment by multiplying the results with a parameter that is close to 1 (and so would not change the score much) to give us the opportunity to slightly lower the score for hitlists obtained from a small database compared to a large one. Because obtaining a short, target-rich hitlist from a larger database is significantly more important than from a small database. (Just as a list of five apartments with high potential, including the three perfect ones for you, in Manhattan is more valuable than a similar list for a small-town housing market.) If the results were obtained from a small database, the multiplier on the right side of the equation would be something like 0.95 instead of 1. Hence, the GH-Score would reduce slightly. But if it were obtained from a large database, the GH-Score would remain high.

A multiplier slightly less than 1 would give a GH-Score selectively reduced in value. If we subtract the $Ht/D$ ratio from 1 (i.e., $1 - Ht/D$), we should be able to make this adjustment to correlate with the database size.

This gives an adjustment as shown below:

$$GH = \left( \frac{Ha \times (3A + Ht)}{4Ht \times A} \right) \times \left( 1 - \frac{Ht}{D} \right)$$

This rendition of the GH-Score worked well, and we started to assess the metric with a best, worst, good, bad, and average hitlist. However, the best hitlist did not give a result of GH = 1 as needed, but a value close to 1 (like 0.999998). Similarly, the score for the worst hitlist came out to be something like 0.000001 instead of GH = 0. This was frustrating, as I wanted the GH score to have a value from 0 to 1. I consulted Dr. Marvin Waldman, who was at Accelrys with me at that time. He looked at my equation for about a minute and said, "Why are you penalizing your score with the count of active compounds?" With that question answered by subtracting the active compounds in the hitlist ($Ht - Ha$), and subtracting the active compounds from the database ($D - A$), we made the final adjustment to account for database size and reached the last version of the GH score:

$$GH = \left( \frac{Ha \times (3A + Ht)}{4Ht \times A} \right) \times \left( 1 - \frac{Ht - Ha}{D - A} \right)$$

...where $Ha$ is the number of active compounds in the hitlist, $Ht$ is the total number of compounds in the hitlist, $D$ is the number of compounds in the database, and $A$ is the number of active compounds in the database.

Now the best hitlist (one retrieving all the active compounds, but nothing but active compound) received the exact score of GH = 1, and the worst hitlist (retrieving all the compounds except the active ones), GH = 0. Mission accomplished!

# APPENDIX IV

- Pharmainformatics: Integration of Bioinformatics and Cheminformatics. 221st ACS, April 2, 2001
- Information Challenges in CombiChem/HTS Era. 222nd ACS, August 28, 2001
- ADME/Tox Informatics (*Chem. Eng. News Cover Story – April 29,2002*), 223rd ACS, April 7-11, 2002
- Virtual High-Throughput Screening. 224th ACS, August 18-22, 2002
- Informatics Challenges in Pharmacogenomics. 225th ACS, March 23-27, 2003
- Advances in Pharmacophores and 3D-Searching. 227th ACS, March 28-31, 2004
- Advances in Virtual High-Throughput Screening. 228th ACS, August 22-26, 2004
- ADME/Tox Informatics. 229th ACS, March 14-20, 2005
- Advances in Data Mining and Analysis: Informatics Perspective. 230th ACS, August 28-30, 2005
- Advances in Data Mining and Analysis: Computational Perspective. 230th ACS, August 28-30, 2005
- Advances in Pharmacophores and 3D Screening. 231st ACS, March 26-30, 200

# APPENDIX V

World Cruise Itinerary
Pacific Princess ® 2016 World Cruise, one hundred and eleven days
January 20, 2016 – May 11, 2016, Round trip from Los Angeles,
   California

| Day | Date | Port |
|---|---|---|
| 1 | Jan 20 | Los Angeles, California |
| 2-6* | Jan 21-25 | Cruising the Pacific Ocean |
| 7 | Jan 26 | Honolulu, Hawaii |
| 8-12 | Jan 27-31 | Cruising the South Pacific Ocean |
|  |  | (Cross the Equator) |
| 13 | Feb 1 | Pago Pago, American Samoa |
| 14 | Feb 2-3 | Cruising the South Pacific Ocean |

| | | |
|---|---|---|
| | | (Cross the International Date Line) |
| 15 | Feb 4 | Nuku'alofa, Tonga |
| 16-17 | Feb 5-6 | Cruising the South Pacific Ocean |
| 18 | Feb 7 | Bay of Islands, New Zealand |
| 19 | Feb 8 | Auckland, New Zealand |
| 20-22 | Feb 9-11 | Cruising the South Pacific Ocean |
| 23 | Feb 12 | Sydney, Australia |
| 24-26 | Feb 13-15 | Cruising the South Pacific Ocean |
| 27 | Feb 16 | Cairns, Australia (for the Great Barrier Reef) |
| 28-30 | Feb 17-19 | Cruising the South Pacific Ocean |
| 31 | Feb 20 | Darwin, Australia |
| 32-35 | Feb 21-24 | Cruising the South Pacific Ocean |
| 36 | Feb 25 | Bandar Seri Begavan (Muara), Brunei |
| 37 | Feb 26 | Kota Kinabalu, Malaysia |

| | | |
|---|---|---|
| 38-39 | Feb 27-28 | Cruising the South China Sea |
| 40 | Feb 29 | Hong Kong |
| 41 | Mar 1 | Hong Kong |
| 42-43 | Mar 2-3 | Cruising the Gulf of Thailand |
| 44 | Mar 4 | Ho Chi Minh City, Viet Nam (Phu My) |
| 45-46 | Mar 5-6 | Cruising the Gulf of Thailand |
| 47 | Mar 7 | Singapore |
| 48-51 | Mar 8-11 | Cruising the Bay of Bengal |
| 52 | Mar 12 | Colombo, Sri Lanka |
| 53 | Mar 13 | Cruising the Indian Ocean |
| 54 | Mar 14 | Mangalore, India |
| 55-56 | Mar 15-16 | Cruising the Indian Ocean |
| 57 | Mar 17 | Muscat, Oman (Mina Qaboos) |
| 58 | Mar 18 | Dubai, United Arab Emirates |
| 59 | Mar 19 | Dubai, United Arab Emirates |

| 60-66 | Mar 20-26 | Cruising the Arabian Sea |
|---|---|---|
| 67 | Mar 27 | Aqaba, Jordan (for Petra) |
| 68 | Mar 28 | Cruising the Red Sea |
| 69 | Mar 29 | Transiting the Suez Canal |
| 70 | Mar 30 | Cruising the Mediterranean Sea |
| 71 | Mar 31 | Rhodes, Greece |
| 72 | Apr 1 | Chania, Crete, Greece |
| 73 | Apr 2 | Cruising the Mediterranean Sea |
| 74 | Apr 3 | Bari, Italy |
| 75 | Apr 4 | Venice, Italy |
| 76 | Apr 5 | Venice, Italy |
| 77 | Apr 6 | Korčula, Croatia |
| 78 | Apr 7 | Cruising the Mediterranean Sea |
| 79 | Apr 8 | Valetta, Malta |
| 80 | Apr 9 | Cruising the Mediterranean Sea |
| 81 | Apr 10 | Palma de Mallorca, Spain |
| 82 | Apr 11 | Cartagena, Spain |

| 83 | Apr 12 | Ceuta, Spanish Morocco |
| 84 | Apr 13 | Cruising the Atlantic Ocean |
| 85 | Apr 14 | Madeira (Funchal), Portugal |
| 86-91 | Apr 15-20 | Cruising the Atlantic Ocean |
| 92 | Apr 21 | Bermuda (Hamilton) |
| 93-94 | Apr 22-23 | Cruising the Atlantic Ocean |
| 95 | Apr 24 | Ft. Lauderdale, Florida |
| 96-97 | Apr 25-26 | Cruising the Caribbean Sea |
| 98 | Apr 27 | Willemstad, Curaçao |
| 99 | Apr 28 | Cruising the Caribbean Sea |
| 100 | Apr 29 | Cartagena, Colombia |
| 101 | Apr 30 | Transiting Panama Canal |
| 102 | May 1 | Cruising the Pacific Ocean |
| 103 | May 2 | Puerto Quepos, Costa Rica |
| 104-106 | May 3-5 | Cruising the Pacific Ocean |

| 107 | May 6 | Puerto Vallarta, Mexico |
| 108 | May 7 | Cruising the Pacific Ocean |
| 109 | May 8 | La Paz, Mexico |
| 110-111 | May 9-10 | Cruising the Pacific Ocean |
| 112 | May 11 | Los Angeles, California |

*Days highlighted with **bold** letters were when the bridge program was delivered

# NOTES

1. ^ You can think of heterocyclic molecules as short pearl necklaces with a ceramic or glass bead or two included in the string; the pearls here stand in for carbon, the other beads for heteroatoms. And you can think of regioisomers as a few of these necklaces with pendants hanging off from different beads in the chain. Stereoisomers, then, would be a few of these necklaces, some with all the pendants pointing above the plane of the flat necklace, and some with pendants pointing either up or down from that plane. Jewelry metaphors aside, organic chemistry requires the skills of an exacting and creative chef more than those of a jeweler, to coax desired outcomes out of complex natural systems—not as easy as picking up the individual pieces and stringing them.

2. ^ Güner, O. F.; Shillady, D. D.; Ottenbrite, R. M.; Rao, B. K.; Yurtsever, E. "Pair-Excitation MCSCF Treatment of Small Molecules in an Optimized Slater-Transform-Preuss (STP) Basis Set." *Int. J. Quantum Chem.* **1987**, *32*, 551-562.

3. ^ A small computer, relative to mainframe computers anyway, and classed as a minicomputer, even though it was still much larger than the not-yet-widely-used PCs.

4. ^ This is similar to how better, more detailed actuarial tables, can better predict the risk that an insuree might file a claim, and such tables are more complicated to decipher than simpler ones.

5. ^ Olah, G. A.; Anizfeld, R.; Prakash, G. H. S.; Williams, R. E.; Lammertsma, K.; Güner, O. F. "Hydrogen-Deuterium Exchange of Diborane in Superacid Solution Through Diboranonium

($B_2H_7^+$), and Diboranium ($B_2H_5^+$) Ions." *J. Am. Chem. Soc.* **1988**, *110*, 7885-7886.

6. ^ Lammertsma, K.; Güner, O. F.; Thibodeaux, A. F.; Schleyer, P. v. R. "Structures and Energies of Isomeric C3H62+ Dications." *J. Am. Chem. Soc.* **1989**, *111*, 8995-9002.

7. ^ Lammertsma, K.; Güner, O. F.; Drewes, R. M.; Reed, A.; Schleyer, P. v. R. "Remarkable Structures of Dialane(4), Al2H4." *Inorg. Chem.* **1989**, *28*, 313-317.

8. ^ The titles of my papers presented at the 196th National Meeting, Los Angeles California were:
"Structural Properties of Tetraatomic $B_2Be_2$ Cluster"
"Protonated Diboranes - A Theoretical Study"
"Hyperconjugative Stabilizations in Carbodications"
"Theoretical Evaluation of Epimerization in Diels-Alder Cycloadducts"

9. ^ The number of citations a paper receives from other scientists in their research is widely considered a valid measure of the paper's influence. Several thousand citations over any time period is *a lot*.

10. ^ Wermuth, C.-G.; Ganellin, C. R.; Lindberg, P.; Mitscher, L. A. Glossary of Terms used in medicinal chemistry (IUPAC recommendations 1998). *Pure Appl. Chem.* **1998**, *70*, 1129–1143.

11. ^ We can classify the general approach to generate pharmacophore models into two categories. If the 3D structure of a receptor and a bound ligand is available, the bound conformation of the ligand can be used to build a model. Appendix I details a stepwise description for this approach. If a 3D structure of a receptor is not available, common patterns among active compounds can provide information to generate pharmacophore models. Similarly, a stepwise description of this approach is also exemplified in Appendix II.

12. ^ Güner, O. F. "The impact of pharmacophores in drug design," *IDrugs,* **2005**, *8*(7), 567-572

13. ^ Güner, O. F.; Dumont, L. M. "3D Searching in Computer-Aided Drug Design." *Pharmaceutical Manufacturers*

*International 1991,* Barber, M.S., Barnacal, P.A., Eds; Sterling Publications: London **1990**; pp 65-68

14. ^ Güner, O. F.; Hughes, D. W.; Dumont, L. M. "An Integrated Approach to Three-Dimensional Information Management with MACCS-3D." *J. Chem. Inf. Comput. Sci.* **1991**, *31*, 408-414.

15. ^ J. J. Kaminski, D. F. Rane, M. E. Snow, L.Weber, M. L. Rothofsky, S. D. Anderson, and S. L. Lin; "Identification of novel farnesyl transferase inhibitors using three-dimensional database searching techniques," *J. Med. Chem.* **1997**, *40*, 25, 4103–4112

16. ^ *Chem. Eng. News* Cover Story – *June 5,* **2000**

17. ^ *Chem. Eng. News* Cover Story – *April 29,* **2002**

18. ^ Pharmacophore Perception, Development, and Use for Drug Design, Osman F. Güner Ed., Int. University Line, La Jolla 2000

19. ^ Güner, O. F. and Henry, D. R. "Metrics for Analyzing Hit Lists and Pharmacophores" in *Pharmacophore Perception, Development, and Use for Drug Design,* Güner, O. F. (Ed.), International University Line, **2000**, 193-211

20. ^ Güner, O. F. Waldman, M.; Hoffmann, R.; Kim, J-H. "Strategies in Database Mining and Pharmacophore Development" in *Pharmacophore Perception, Development, and Use for Drug Design,* Güner, O. F. (Ed.), International University Line, **2000**, 213-232.

21. ^ Raymond, J.W. and Willett, P., "Effectiveness of graph-based and fingerprint-based similarity measures for virtual screening of 2D chemical structure databases" *J. Comp.-Aided Molec. Des.,* **2002**, *16(1)*, 59-71.

22. ^ The database construction need not only convert two-dimensional structures into 3D conformations, but also to address issues around tautomerism, stereochemistry, conformational flexibility, and ionization states.

23. ^ Bowen, J. P.; Güner, O. F. "A Perspective on Quantum Mechanics Calculations in ADMET Predictions" *Curr. Top. Med. Chem.,* **2013**, *13*(11), 1257-1272.

24. ^ Güner, O. F.; Bowen, J. P. "Pharmacophore Modeling for ADME" *Curr. Top. Med. Chem.,* **2013**, *13*(11), 1327-1342.

25. ^ Güner, O. F.; Bowen, J. P. "Setting the Record Straight: The Origin of the Pharmacophore Concept" *J. Chem. Inf. Model.,* **2014**, *54* (5), 1269–1283.

26. ^ The fact that Dr. Ehrlich had never used the term pharmacophore does not mean that he did not develop the concept. A more recent example for a similar scenario is that Albert Einstein is credited for developing of the concept of photons in his famous 1905 paper, yet he never used the term himself (he referred to it as "energy quanta"). Gilbert Lewis introduced the name "photon" many years later in 1926. Even after that, to my knowledge, Einstein refused to use the term in his publications and presentations.

27. ^ Murnane, K. S.; Güner, O. F.; Bowen, J. P; Rambacher, K. M.; Moniri, N. H,; Murphy, T. J.; Daphney, C. M.; Oppong-Damoah, A.; Rice. K. C., "The adrenergic receptor antagonist carvedilol interacts with serotonin 2A receptors both *in vitro* and *in vivo,*" *Pharmacology, Biochemistry and Behavior,* **2019**, *181,* 37–45.

28. ^ A pathway is simply a stepwise series of biochemical reactions to achieve a certain biological outcome, with specific molecules playing a role at each step. Molecules called enzymes speed those reactions along.

29. ^ Phosphorylation is the transfer of phosphate molecule to the enzyme, essentially readying it for action.

30. ^ Uko, N. E.; Güner, O. F.; Barnett, L. M. A.; Matesic, D. F.; Bowen, J. P. "Discovery and biological activity of computer-assisted drug designed Akt pathway inhibitors," *Bioorg. Med. Chem. Lett,* **2018**, *28,* 3247-3250.

31. ^ Uko, N. E.; Güner, O. F.; Bowen, J. P.; Matesic, D. F. "Akt Pathway Inhibition of the Solenopsin Analog, 2-Dodecyl-sulfanyl-1,-4,-5,-6-tetrahydropyrimidine," *Anticancer Research,* **2019**, *39,* 5329-5338.

32. ^ Uko N.E.; Güner O.F.; Matesic D.F.; Bowen J.P. "Akt Pathway Inhibitors," *Curr. Top. Med. Chem.* **2020**, *20*(10), 883-900.

33. ^ Phillips, R. S.; Anderson, A. D.; Gentry, H. G.; Güner, O. F.; Bowen, J. P. "Substrate and inhibitor specificity of kynurenine monooxygenase from *Cytophaga hutchinsonii*", *Bioorg. Med. Chem. Lett.,* **2017**, *27*(8), 1705-1708.

34. ^ Hughes, T.D.; Güner, O.F.; Iradukunda, E.C.; Phillips, R.S.; Bowen J.P. " The Kynurenine Pathway and Kynurenine 3-Monooxygenase Inhibitors," *Molecules*, **2022**, *27*(273), 1-26.

35. ^ Xu, Q.; Kulkarni, A. A.; Meleveetil, S.; Hussein, D.; Brown, D.; Güner, O. F.; Reddy, M. D.; Watkins, E. B.; Lassègue, B.; Griendling, K. K.; Bowen, J. P. "Design, synthesis, and biological evaluation of inhibitors of the NADPH oxidase, Nox4," *Bioorg. Med. Chem.,* **2018**, *26*, 989-998.

36. ^ Watkins, E. B.; Güner, O. F.; Kulkarni, A.; Lassègue, B.; Griendling, K. K.; Bowen, J. P. "Discovery and Therapeutic Relevance of Small-Molecule NOX4 Inhibitors," *Med. Chem. Rev.,* **2018**, *53*(8), 135-150.

37. ^ Güner, O. F. *et al.*, "NADPH Oxidase Inhibitors and Uses Thereof," US Patent: US2020/0270214 A1

38. ^ The duplicate bridge game, the standard competitive game, allows teams to play the same hands with identical decks and compare the results against all the other teams who played the same hands.